THE LANGUAGE OF TRAUMA

War and Technology in Hoffmann, Freud, and Kafka

From the Napoleonic Wars to the invention of the railway to the shell shock of World War I, writers tried to give voice to the suffering that war and industrial technology had wrought all around them. Yet they, like the doctors who treated these victims, repeatedly ran up against the incapacity of language to describe such anguish; those who suffered trauma, those who tried to heal it, and those who represented it were all unable to find the appropriate words. In *The Language of Trauma*, John Zilcosky uncovers the reactions of three major central European writers – E.T.A. Hoffmann, Sigmund Freud, and Franz Kafka – to the birth of modern trauma in the nineteenth and early twentieth centuries.

Zilcosky makes the case that Hoffmann, Freud, and Kafka managed to find the language of trauma precisely by *not* attempting to name the trauma conclusively and instead allowing their writing to mimic the experience itself. Just as the victims' symptoms seemed not to correspond to a physical cause, the writers' words did not connect directly to the objects of the world. While doctors attempted to overcome this indeterminacy, these writers embraced and investigated it; they sought a language that described language's tragic limits and that, in so doing, exemplified the wider literary and philosophical crisis of their time. Zilcosky boldly argues that this linguistic scepticism emerged together with the medical inability to name the experience of trauma. He thereby places trauma where it belongs: at the heart of both medicine's diagnostic predicament and modern literature's most daring experiments.

JOHN ZILCOSKY is a professor of German and Comparative Literature at the University of Toronto.

The Language of Trauma

War and Technology in Hoffmann, Freud, and Kafka

JOHN ZILCOSKY

UNIVERSITY OF TORONTO PRESS
Toronto Buffalo London

University of Toronto Press
Toronto Buffalo London
utorontopress.com

ISBN 978-1-4875-0939-2 (cloth)   ISBN 978-1-4875-0941-5 (EPUB)
ISBN 978-1-4875-0942-2 (paper)   ISBN 978-1-4875-0940-8 (PDF)

Library and Archives Canada Cataloguing in Publication

Title: The language of trauma : war and technology in Hoffmann,
Freud, and Kafka / John Zilcosky.
Names: Zilcosky, John, author.
Description: Includes bibliographical references and index.
Identifiers: Canadiana (print) 20210153261 | Canadiana (ebook)
20210153415 | ISBN 9781487509392 (cloth) | ISBN 9781487509422
(paper) | ISBN 9781487509415 (EPUB) | ISBN 9781487509408 (PDF)
Subjects: LCSH: Hoffmann, E. T. A. (Ernst Theodor Amadeus),
1776–1822. Sandmann. | LCSH: Freud, Sigmund, 1856–1939.
Unheimliche. | LCSH: Kafka, Franz, 1883–1924. Verwandlung. |
LCSH: Psychic trauma in literature. | LCSH: European literature –
History and criticism.
Classification: LCC PN56.P914 Z55 2021 | DDC 809/.93353–dc23

This book has been published with the help of a grant from the Federation
for the Humanities and Social Sciences, through the Awards to Scholarly
Publications Program, using funds provided by the Social Sciences and
Humanities Research Council of Canada.

University of Toronto Press acknowledges the financial assistance to its
publishing program of the Canada Council for the Arts and the Ontario Arts
Council, an agency of the Government of Ontario.

Canada Council   Conseil des Arts
for the Arts   du Canada

ONTARIO ARTS COUNCIL
CONSEIL DES ARTS DE L'ONTARIO
an Ontario government agency
un organisme du gouvernement de l'Ontario

Funded by the   Financé par le
Government   gouvernement
of Canada   du Canada

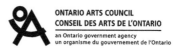

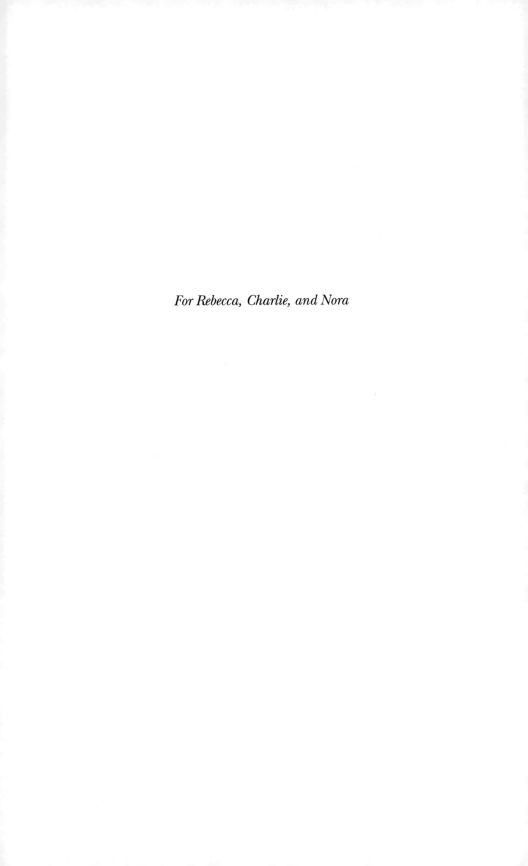

For Rebecca, Charlie, and Nora

Contents

Illustrations

Acknowledgments

It is a joy to remember all the people who helped me over the years of writing this book. For financial support, I thank the Alexander von Humboldt Foundation, whose Friedrich-Wilhelm-Bessel Research Prize allowed me to spend a semester in Berlin completing my research. The Foundation – personified for me by Katrin Amian, Maria-Bernadette Carstens-Behrens, and Steffen Mehlich – big-heartedly helped my family to set down roots in Berlin. I am grateful to the director of Berlin's Leibniz-Zentrum für Literatur- und Kulturforschung (ZfL), Eva Geulen, who welcomed me and gave me the opportunity to deliver a public lecture. I thank especially my host, Stefan Willer, who integrated me in the life of the ZfL and, a year later, invited me to the Humboldt University to present further research. I remember too the expert librarians at the Staatsbibliothek zu Berlin (especially the E.T.A.-Hoffmann-Archiv) and the archivists at the Humboldt University Archive, which holds the records for the Charité Hospital's Clinic for Nervous Diseases.

For their invitations to present drafts of this book publicly, I thank Wolfgang Asholt (Cerisy), Cathy Caruth (Cornell), Stanley Corngold (Princeton), Kata Gellen and Saskia Ziolkowski (Duke), Jason Lieblang and Ilinca Iurascu (University of British Columbia), and Robert Stockhammer (Munich). Some of the ideas in this book were hatched in briefer article form, where they benefited from the generous advice of the editors of *Kafka for the Twenty-First Century* and *Psychoanalysis and History*. I am grateful also to Wolf Kittler for co-organizing with me a three-day seminar on war trauma at the German Studies Association Conference in Kansas City. There I met Paul Lerner, who shared with me his insights on the history of German psychiatry. Christine Lehleiter, Matt Ffytche, Ritchie Robertson, and André Flicker also offered valuable suggestions. I gained inspiration from the smart and passionate students in my comparative literature graduate seminar, "Literature, Trauma, Modernity." Len Husband at the University of Toronto Press loved this project from the beginning and spurred me on; the savvy Anne Laughlin and Christine Robertson expertly guided me to the finish line. My brilliant research assistants, Maral Attar-Zadeh and Mikaela Kennedy, helped at every step of the way.

Finally, I am grateful to my wife, Rebecca, and our children, Charlie and Nora, who hunkered down sportingly with me through the pandemic – tolerating my disappearances into my study, even though, as Charlie reminded me, I do not really "have to" write books anymore. For better or for worse, I wrote this one, and I dedicate it to them.

Abbreviations

Hoffmann

SW   *Sämtliche Werke*
Dv   "Drei verhängnisvolle Monate!," in SW 1:802–8
S   "The Sandman," in *Tales of Hoffmann*, 85–125
Sg   "Der Sandmann," in SW 3:11–49
T   "Tagebuch 1813," in SW 1:442–88
V   "Die Vision auf dem Schlachtfelde bei Dresden," in SW
      2.1:479–82

Freud

GW   *Gesammelte Werke*
SE   *Standard Edition*
F   *Complete Letters of Freud to Fliess*
Fg   *Briefe an Wilhelm Fließ*
U   "The Uncanny," in SE 17:217–56
Ug   "Das Unheimliche," in GW 12:229–68

Kafka

AS   *Amtliche Schriften*
BF   *Briefe an Felice*
B   *Briefe 1902–24*
CS   *The Complete Stories*
Di   *Diaries 1910–23*
D   *Drucke zu Lebzeiten*
K   *Kafka's Selected Stories*
L   *Letters to Friends, Family, and Editors*
LF   *Letters to Felice*
M   *The Metamorphosis*
MP   *The Metamorphosis, the Penal Colony, and Other Stories*
N   *Nachgelassene Schriften und Fragmente*, 2 volumes (N1 and N2)
O   *Blue Octavo Notebooks*

Note on Translations

Where reliable English translations exist for Hoffmann, Freud, and Kafka, I cite from them – emending where necessary (including, in those cases, the original German). When no translation is mentioned, the translation is my own.

THE LANGUAGE OF TRAUMA

War and Technology in Hoffmann, Freud, and Kafka

Literature, Trauma, and the Sign of Illness

The idea for this book came to me over twenty years ago, while I was reading popular travel journals from around 1900 for my first book, *Kafka's Travels*. I was searching for descriptions of why people travelled, specifically of the travellers' dreams, fantasies, and aspirations. But I kept coming across discussions of travel's dangers – caused mostly by trains – and discovered that fin-de-siècle travellers and physicians were obsessed with the illnesses caused by these racing masses of steel. Although these pathologies of the railway never found their way into *Kafka's Travels*, they left me wondering how much Kafka knew about them and, more than this, whether they played a role in his decision to make his famously "ill" modernist protagonist, Gregor Samsa, a professional train traveller. Years later, I researched Kafka's work in accident insurance as well as his own anxieties about trains and found astounding similarities between Samsa and the victims of so-called *Eisenbahnkrankheiten* (railway illnesses). The language of trauma from Kafka's day, it turned out, had made its marks on his apparently otherworldly hero.

This discovery of contemporaneous trauma discourse in a novella otherwise known for its existentialist refusal of the real world led me to consider similar examples in modernism and romanticism. James Joyce's *Ulysses* (1922), the prototypical modernist novel, has traditionally been read as transcending the historical actuality of its streets, pubs, and landmarks in 1904 Dublin. Scholars emphasize the novel's investigation of deep psychological experience through stream-of-consciousness style and this experience's rootedness in

myth. The Greek/Roman protagonist, Odysseus/Ulysses, reappears
as the modern Everyman, Leopold Bloom. Bloom makes his way
home from Glasnevin Cemetery just as Odysseus travelled back
from Troy and Hades. For T.S. Eliot, this "mythic method" allowed
Joyce to distance himself from his contemporary world and, in so
doing, create a transcendent modernism. Deconstructionist readers
from the 1970s onward took this anti-realist claim further: *Ulysses* is
not even primarily about myth but about the lack of historical reference altogether. The novel's playful use of language and its shifting
styles reveal that its major concern is literature itself – specifically,
language's ironic tendency to refer back only to language.

This anti-referential reading of *Ulysses* carried over to the traditional history of the novel's composition, particularly as it relates
to World War I. Joyce began *Ulysses* in Trieste in 1914, the year the
war started, and published its first excerpt in 1918, the year the war
ended. He completed *Ulysses*'s first three episodes in 1917, on the
heels of the bloody 1916 battles of Verdun and the Somme – during
which the magnitude and brutality of the war became clear to all.
Shortly before this, Joyce had moved to neutral Switzerland, where
the myth of his own private "neutrality" was born. While the British
fought the Germans in Passchendaele, he hid himself away in Zurich and Locarno – "kuskykorked himself up tight in his inkbattle
house" – where he wrote about the Dublin of his youth.[1] As Richard Ellmann claims in the classic biography of Joyce that has long
defined the story of *Ulysses*'s genesis, Switzerland embodied Joyce's
political disinterest: it was "more than a refuge; it was a symbol of
artistic detachment, *au-dessus de la mêlée.*"[2]

But more recent critics have given the lie to this myth, demon-
strating that, although Joyce never mentions the war in *Ulysses*, the
novel is saturated with it. *Ulysses*, it turns out, is shot through with
hidden war references, especially in the "Nestor" chapter, which
Joyce completed in autumn 1917. Stephen Daedalus lectures on the
ancient Greek general Pyrrhus, whose "Another victory like that and
we're done for" recalled contemporaneous quips about the British
"victory" on the Somme. Here and throughout *Ulysses*, we see significant traces of the hostilities and even, as Robert Spoo wrote already
in 1986, a comprehensive "inscribing of the nightmare of war within

the ostensible neutrality of the 1904 narrative."[3] Peter Barham, one of the recent scholars to recognize Spoo's point and tie *Ulysses* to the war, begins several chapters and subchapters of his 2004 book about shell shock, *Forgotten Lunatics of the Great War*, with epigraphs from Joyce's novel. *Ulysses*, he argues, is "a war novel *par excellence*"; it "is permeated by the war without once mentioning it."[4] This novel, apparently about language's self-referentiality and the myth of the Trojan War, turns out also to be about the war of its own time, as it raged around its author.

Ulysses is not the only apparently hermetic modernist work that is troubled by the war and its traumas. Most obvious are Virginia Woolf's 1925 *Mrs. Dalloway* and Marcel Proust's *In Search of Lost Time* (1913–27). The former, like *Ulysses*, describes one day in the inner lives of ordinary people but ends up being haunted by the memories of a shell-shocked veteran. *In Search of Lost Time* similarly focuses on the psychic interiors of aristocratic France, for thousands of pages, until German Zeppelin raids and the blackout of Paris intrude in the final volume. Less apparent is Thomas Mann's 1924 *The Magic Mountain*, whose relation to the war is actually closest to *Ulysses*.[5] Like *Ulysses*, *The Magic Mountain* takes place in the prelapsarian world before the war and thus seems to have nothing to do with it; yet, like *Ulysses*, it was written partially during the hostilities, which left unmistakable traces on it. The war appears anachronistically in *The Magic Mountain* even more directly than in *Ulysses*. According to *The Magic Mountain*'s plot, the war has not yet begun, but the protagonist's dead cousin reappears, bearing marks of that war, towards the end of the novel. He materializes in a séance wearing a World War I uniform and the iconic steel helmet – *Stahlhelm* – that the Germans did not even begin producing until 1916. What is more, this cousin, like Woolf's Septimus Smith, bears the typical wounds and expression of a World War I shell-shock victim.[6]

Another classic modernist work that seemed to have little to do with the war (beyond a passing mention of demobbing) is Eliot's *The Waste Land* (1922). But it too turns out to contain hidden references to war and shock. For Peter Middleton, the poem is actually "a response to the war."[7] Maud Ellmann builds on this claim, arguing that *The Waste Land* reveals "the specific absence that succeeded

World War I" and "evinces both the dread and the desire to hear the voices" of the dead and injured soldiers.[8] Such concealed markers of war and trauma are not limited to modernism. Already in the supposedly hermetic nineteenth-century poetry of Emily Dickinson (1830–1886), for example, we see this poetry's "objective counterpart in physical and palpable warfare": the carnage of the American Civil War.[9]

With this group of seemingly self-enclosed modern texts in mind, my first, more modest, goal is to add other works that are likewise quietly permeated by war and by industrial trauma – especially that associated with travel by railway. For this, I have chosen exemplary writings: from romanticism (E.T.A. Hoffmann's "The Sandman"), from modernism's crossover genre of fiction mixed with science or philosophy (Freud's "strange theoretical novel," *The Uncanny*),[10] and from literary modernism itself (Kafka's *The Metamorphosis* as well as his late stories). In each of these cases, I engage in close readings to reveal the contemporaneous discourse of trauma that has, till now, remained concealed: in "The Sandman," the Napoleonic Wars; in *The Uncanny*, shell shock from World War I; in Kafka's *The Metamorphosis*, the pathology of the railway journey; and in his late stories, the trauma caused precisely by the desire to have one's trauma recognized. Medical researchers referred to this desire as "pension neurosis" – a neurosis created by the longing for a pension – and later as "pension-struggle neurosis" (*Rentenkampfneurose*): a neurosis caused by the stress of trying to convince the bureaucracy to release one's pension. This bureaucratic catch-22 indeed plagues many of Kafka's characters.

My second, more ambitious, goal is to connect this medical language of trauma with the language of scepticism in romanticism and modernism, specifically, through the two discourses' obsession with inscrutability. The modern science of trauma – issuing from the nineteenth-century concurrence of industrial violence and medical empiricism – faced a particularly hermeneutic, "literary" problem. Weeks after surviving a battle or a railway accident, patients presented a baffling series of symptoms: sobbing, shaking, twitching, sleeplessness, blurred vision, and so on. Because doctors could find no physical source to which these symptoms pointed, they invented one. During the Napoleonic Wars (1803–15), for example, they concocted the *vent du boulet* (wind-of-the-cannonball or "wind-contusion") syndrome, claiming that symptomatic yet uninjured soldiers had suffered inner ear injuries when cannonballs had whizzed past them.

During the period of massive railway expansion that began in the 1860s and 1870s, doctors argued that their mysteriously ill patients had injured their spines during collisions or through the continual shaking and jolting of the trains ("railway spine"). After autopsies of spines revealed no damage, researchers from the 1880s and 1890s shifted their focus to the brain. A "molecular rearrangement" in the cerebral cortex must have pathologically affected "the centers for motility, sensitiveness, and sensate functions"; this "railway-brain" theory had many supporters into World War I.[11] But because this molecular source remained "submicroscopic," the theory did not solve the problem of locating a physical source.[12] Instead it created only further uncertainty; neither patient nor doctor could see or touch the source of suffering. The physical lesion that was supposed to be the symptom's underlying truth now became its anxiogenic missing origin.

This "ultramodern" hermeneutical language of the "undetectable pathological-anatomical substrate" dovetailed with the linguistic scepticism of the literature and philosophy of the period.[13] Whether we begin in the early nineteenth century with the playwright Heinrich von Kleist's "Kant crisis" – his despair over our inability to access "truth"[14] – or romantic irony's general sense that the literary text referred primarily to itself, we see a growing suspicion, from 1800 onward, that words could not describe a world beyond themselves. Nietzsche drove this suspicion to its logical extreme in *On Truth and Lie in an Extra-Moral Sense* (1873) and *Human All Too Human* (1878–80), insisting that language was defined by nothing other than its unreliability.[15] Language was inherently unable to say what it wanted to; it always "lied." This scepticism developed into a crisis around 1900, through the poets of *Sprachskepsis*. I think of Stefan George or of Rainer Maria Rilke, who was "filled with fear" in 1899 by "the words of humans" (*vor der Menschen Wort*). Hugo von Hofmannsthal similarly wrote in his 1902 "Chandos" letter that

words were "whirlpools [*Wirbel*] ... reeling incessantly," which caused
Chandos to suffer "vertigo" and the sensation of falling into "the
void."[16] Simultaneously, Fritz Mauthner issued a Nietzsche-inspired
philosophical tract on the unreliability of language: the two-volume
Contributions to a Critique of Language (1901–2), which eventually became important to Wittgenstein.

In 1906, the linguist Ferdinand de Saussure began his famous
Course in General Linguistics, in which he examined the instability
of all linguistic signs. The sign, he argued, was split. It consisted of
the signifier (the written or spoken word) and the signified (the
concept or object towards which the signifier pointed). The relation between these two was "arbitrary," Saussure contended, in that
there was no "natural connection" between, say, the letters C-A-T
and the furry four-legged creature to which these supposedly referred.[17] Saussure's insights deepened the crisis of signification –
leading eventually to Claude Lévi-Strauss's claim that signifiers can
"float" over and above the content of a particular signified,[18] and to
poststructuralism's vaunted insistence on the signifier's "free play."

The nineteenth- and early twentieth-century discourses of medical
trauma and of language scepticism converged in this disconnection of
the signifier from the signified. Although medical researchers never
stated this, they knew implicitly that medical symptoms resembled linguistic signs. The traditional German word for symptom tells us as
much: "Krankheits*zeichen*," the "*sign* of illness." More precisely, the
symptom corresponds to the sign's "signifier," whereas the pathological anatomical substrate, or cause, is its "signified." For many non-trau-
matic nineteenth-century illnesses, this medical semiotics seemed to
work. Even if researchers had not yet discovered a cure for tuberculosis, for example, they were relatively sure that the symptom (chronic
coughing, often of sputum and blood) linked to an anatomical substrate (a lesion on the lung); this could be proven through autopsies.
And following Robert Koch's 1882 discovery of *M. tuberculosis*, physicians could point to a specific bacterium in the patient's body that
could be isolated and observed through a microscope. But the new
"uninjured" bodies suffering from the traumatic effects of modern
weapons and vehicles resisted this medical semiotics. The symptom
no longer referred to a physical substrate. To use Saussure's words,

the relation between the two had become undependable, apparently "arbitrary." The symptom, like the signifier, seemed to "float."

If we can speak in this way of a hermeneutic crisis in the medical history of trauma, can we likewise speak of a traumatic form of narration in romanticism and modernism? The trauma of trains and war appears in the subtexts of nineteenth- and early twentieth-century literature, and more important, these traumas affect the authors' ways of telling stories. In Hoffmann's "The Sandman," for example, as I discuss in chapter 1, the trauma that Hoffmann witnessed at the 1813 Battle of Dresden forms an uncanny subplot. Hoffmann's narrator in "The Sandman" watches his friend die from a "shattered head" just as Hoffmann, two years earlier, had watched a soldier get hit by a grenade and die from a "shattered head." But more important, the traumatic style from Hoffmann's war diaries transfers to his story. "The Sandman's" narrator zooms in and out of his protagonist's head just as Hoffmann did with the participants in the battle, blurring the relation between the narrator's "I" and the character's "he." And after the narrator witnesses the violent death, he responds with a dash that fills "several years": an abrupt caesura that is the stylistic marker of repression.

My second chapter focuses on Freud's *The Uncanny* (1919), a prototypical modernist crossover text on a par with Nietzsche's *Thus Spake Zarathrusta*, Oscar Wilde's *De Profundis*, and Walter Benjamin's *Berlin Childhood*. Freud's curiosity about "The Sandman" incited *The Uncanny*, and like its predecessor, *The Uncanny* contains an undiscovered subtext about war: that of World War I. We discover in *The Uncanny* hidden references to soldiers buried alive in the trenches, to a traumatized soldier returning from colonial New Guinea, and to a series of shaking, amputated bodies that mimicked the shell-shocked veterans on Europe's streets. The fact that Freud never named these victims creates an uncanny effect within the text itself, making it a traumatic narrative twice over: it stages the same "return of the repressed" that Freud diagnosed and also demonstrates how the concealed symptoms of shock, like the floating signs of trauma within *The Uncanny*, peregrinate contagiously from subject to subject. This effect infects the style of the text, whose authority is undone by an erratic mixture of evidence, legend, and personal anecdote. Within this, the perspective shifts from the objective third person of science to the first person of "Freud," who becomes a fragile character in his own "strange theoretical novel." He is the "elderly gentleman" spooked on a night train, susceptible to the same hysterical contagion that threatened the war veterans.

In my third chapter, I examine Kafka's *The Metamorphosis*, written in 1912, as well as the stories he composed from the middle of World War I till his death in 1924. The protagonist of *The Metamorphosis*, Gregor Samsa, is a travelling salesman who bears the marks of fin-de-siècle "railway illness." In Gregor's self-diagnosis, he is suffering from an "occupational ailment of the traveling salesman" (M 7). But, more important, Gregor suffers from the diagnostic indeterminability of his illness. Like the traumas that Kafka knew from the Balkan Wars that began just before he started writing this novella, Gregor's illness produces symptoms that can "no longer be traced back to their causes" (18). Gregor thus fears the "insurance doctor": both because this doctor will assume that he is faking and also because Gregor himself cannot know whether the doctor might in fact be right (5). This undecidability is also at the heart of Kafka's style: his unravelling of rhetorical figures, especially metaphor, to demonstrate the indeterminacy of language. He produces here a master metaphor that is always labile, in motion, leaving us forever wondering: Is Gregor a bug or "our" son? At the same time, Kafka creates a character who, like the insurance doctor, can never really know whether he is ill. The scholarly axiom that Gregor's body is a "free-floating" signifier now appears in a new light,[19] as part and parcel of medicine's own semiotic crisis.

In Kafka's late stories (1917–24), which I analyse at the end of this chapter, this problem of semiotic dysfunction intensifies. Written after Kafka was given responsibility for determining whether war veterans were worthy of pensions,[20] these stories reflect the "battle over simulation" (*Simulationsstreit*) waged in Kafka's own medical-insurance industry:[21] If a symptom has no anatomical counterpart, is the patient even ill? The boy in "A Country Doctor" calls for the "government doctor" to confirm that he is "really" sick (K 64). The protagonist of "A Little Woman" exhibits what Kafka calls "Krankheitszeichen," and her neighbour thinks that these are faked (D 326). But what is this neighbour to do when he, like the figures in Freud's *The Uncanny*, begins to contract the same ones? The protagonist of "Josefine, the Singer" unconvincingly claims that she is ill, and her countrymen do not believe her. They sense that she is simulating her fits of fainting and crying to be exempted from work. But they ultimately admit that they have no idea why she is sobbing; her tears are "inexplicable" (K 107). This mystery pertains here even more powerfully than in *The Metamorphosis*, for Josefine and the other late protagonists live in a premodern world where there is not even the possibility of an industrial cause. Kafka decapitates the symptom fully from the cause, just as he completely separates the metaphor's vehicle from its tenor. Only through this decoupling can he investigate the "despair" in language's "helpless[ness]" – and construct his traumatic poetics, based on this brokenness of illness's "sign" (Di 398).

Because I aim to unearth such repressed, formal effects of trauma, I do not discuss the obvious: the nineteenth- and early twentieth-century masterpieces that directly described the traumas of war and technology. To name just a few: *War and Peace* delineates how the Napoleonic Wars created debilitating traumas that seemed to have no basis in physical injury. Charles Dickens exposes the deleterious effects of train travel in *Dombey and Son* and in his late stories, right after Dickens himself was traumatized by a railway accident. And Ernst Jünger describes in *Storm of Steel* the uncanniness of technological warfare in World War I: the brutalizing shells seem to appear out of nowhere, as a manifestation of ghosts (*eine gespenstische Erscheinung*).[22] One could also cite, relating specifically to the railways, the 1880s poems and plays of the German realists and naturalists: Theodor Fontane's "Bridge on the Tay" and Gerhardt Hauptmann's "In the Night Train" and *Signalman Thiel*.

Regarding World War I, the list is long, but begins with – in addition to the memoirs by Jünger and Robert Graves – *A Farewell to Arms, Im Westen Nichts Neues* (*All Quiet on the Western Front*), *Memoirs of an Infantry Officer*, and *Le Feu* (*Under Fire*). I do not mean to imply that these novels are free of the formal literary crisis that I am analysing in romanticism and modernism. But I have chosen texts that do not directly address war and modern technology because, precisely in their silence around any actual event, they engage with trauma on a secondary level. They thus recreate the semiotic crisis at the heart of the medical trauma discourse. Moreover, they perform that crisis in a peculiar way of writing history – an anti-history. They precisely do *not* name history's equivalent for the anatomical substrate: the "real" causal occurrence at the heart of traditional historiography.

This literary resistance, which brings up the larger problem of causality that I am addressing here, generates obvious questions. Am I suggesting, for example, that this traumatic literary narration develops *because* of the indeterminability central to medical diagnostics? On the one hand, yes, for I am indeed claiming that Hoffmann, Kafka, and Freud reacted to the traumas – and corresponding crises in medical discourses – created by the Napoleonic Wars, train travel, the Balkan Wars, and World War I. But in a more complex sense, the answer is no, or at least not yes in a straightforward way.

This complication is necessary because one cannot speak of "medical" and "literary/philosophical" discourses as if they were two separate things. As Mark Micale argues, these two worlds were much closer in the nineteenth and early twentieth centuries than they are today. Owing to a common humanistic education and "pool of cultural resources," scientists and writers shared concepts and vocabularies. Physicians read widely in philosophy and art, and novelists and philosophers incorporated the "findings of medical science" into their work.[23] Towering examples are the physician and dramatist Arthur Schnitzler, a friend of Freud's, and of course Freud himself, who never won a Nobel Prize for medicine but earned the Goethe Prize for his prose.

This blurring of medical and humanistic discourses expressed itself powerfully in the problem of causality. The very idea that doctors should find an anatomical source for a traumatic symptom sprang initially from humanistic thinking. From the late seventeenth century onward, philosophical empiricists such as John Locke and David Hume had attacked the Aristotelian theory of causality, with its assumption of a noumenal source; they argued instead for a logical causality based on strictly observable phenomena. This laid the groundwork for a new empiricism in medicine that discarded essentialist claims – that a balance of invisible humours determined health or illness. One of these modern practitioners was Xavier Bichat, whose *Anatomie générale* (1801) led to the anatomo-clinical method, which claimed that clinical signs were linked to anatomical lesions.[24] This could be proven through autopsy, using the protocols developed in the 1840s by Rudolf Virchow. The invention of the compound microscope by Zeiss and the introduction of the science of bacteriology by Koch cemented this method, which Jean-Martin Charcot applied to neurology (using autopsies of the spine and brain) and later, in the 1880s, to hysteria.[25] This positivistic approach to trauma's etiologies, with its necessary failures, had a powerful effect on the writers and thinkers I discuss in this book. And these humanists in turn reinfluenced the scientists, not least through crossover figures such as Schnitzler and Freud – who studied with Charcot – as well as Ernst Mach, whose writing blurred the lines between physics, philosophy, and psychology.

On the topic of causality, Mach is the best example of disciplinary border-crossing. Like the classical philosophical empiricists, Mach favoured phenomenological over essentialist causality. But in reaction to increasingly rigid forms of nineteenth-century positivism,[26] he began to question the ground of causality in general. He replaced the term "cause and effect" in 1905 with a sense-based system of "function" or "relation," through the image of a "multiple chain" of "simultaneous and reversible dependences." To describe these dependences, he employed the romantic, anti-causal concept of "coherence" or "connection" (*Zusammenhang*).[27] Not surprisingly, this idea inspired literary modernists, especially the Germans and Austrians – Kafka, Schnitzler, Robert Musil, and Hugo von Hofmannsthal – who knew Mach from his famous professorial tenures in Prague and Vienna.[28] But Mach's theory also influenced scientists such as Freud and Einstein (who wrote an obituary for Mach), as well as medical researchers. These medical researchers began to question the very existence of the "determinate cause" that had been so central to positivistic diagnostics throughout the nineteenth century. As I discuss in my conclusion, such physicians ultimately wondered whether their patients' symptoms could be traced to any cause at all or only to a nebulously intertwined group of "conditions."[29] With Mach as the common denominator between science and medicine on the one hand and literature and philosophy on the other, we see how a modern theory of causality itself cannot be traced back to an original discipline, much less a particular source.

Because literary romanticism and modernism – like Mach's philosophy – proffer criticisms of causality, they can hardly be woven into a straightforward intellectual history. Modern literature destroys the traditional sign and refuses to name causal events, thereby undermining determinate ways of writing the history of trauma. Kafka makes this point when discussing Gregor Samsa's physical transformation in *The Metamorphosis.* It is difficult, if not impossible, Gregor says, to trace things "back to their causes." This insight guides the methodology of my book. Although the causal crisis in the medical diagnosis of trauma does incite literary reactions, the opposite occurs as well. We can speak best, like Mach, of reversible and "multiple" dependences, or with the romantics themselves of *Zusammenhang* – of this condition that, as Walter Benjamin argues, is never "simply causal."[30] For although medical and literary discourses are intertwined, as revealed in the literary texts I discuss here, the literary texts demolish strict causalities. If they point to any historical causes, these are undermined in the moment of gesturing. Yet at the same time this undoing itself points towards a historical truth: the broken semiotics of trauma.

My argument about the relation between modern literature and the medical history of trauma is meant to be neither comprehensive nor conclusive. I aim to make a bold theoretical intervention that allows for new ways of looking at modern literature from the perspective of a crisis in the semiotics of traumatic illness. To put it succinctly, my goal is twofold. First, I aim to delineate how those who suffered from trauma, those who tried to heal it, and those who represented it searched for a language that would explain and give voice to the suffering. Second, I want to reveal how this quest for a language of trauma defined a broader cultural crisis that extended across medical and literary discourses.

The similarities and differences between these discourses are at the heart of my book. Medical doctors and literary authors tried to develop a new way of speaking about trauma, with doctors focusing on a language of explanation and writers seeking a language of expression. Yet Freud uniquely created a form of writing that encompassed both. And, as I argue here, Hoffmann and Kafka did likewise. They constructed figures like Nathanael and Gregor to explain traumatic suffering *and* let it speak. Like actual trauma victims, these protagonists suffer from what doctors termed "multiple" or "agglutinated" causes,[31] and this accumulation increases their suffering. What Freud called overdetermination intersects here with indeterminacy. Just as condensed Freudian dream elements refer to sundry unconscious sources, so too do the symptoms of Nathanael and Gregor point to countless causes – none of which seems to account fully for their symptoms. Nathanael's "utter melancholy" stems from his childhood, his present, and his author's past; its Ur-scene is his home, his mind, and a distant battlefield; and its originator is a "sandman" who is at once his father, an evil stranger, and the mythical "tyrant" Napoleon (S 85, V 479). Gregor's tragic transformation likewise has too many sources: train travel, an unloving family, an alienated life, and most of all, the uncertainty that this mishmash of sources produces. The overdetermined metaphor of Gregor's body becomes the poetic image that expresses the indeterminate suffering of trauma.

Further research might find these same traumatic metaphors lurking in similarly self-referential, sceptical romantic and modernist texts – perhaps also in visual art. Many of these works seem initially, like the ones discussed here, to be disconnected from the catastrophes of war and industrialization. I think of Hölderlin, Wordsworth, and Poe in the romantic era, and of Woolf, Valéry, and Wallace Stevens in the modernist period. But reconfigurations of Woolf's Septimus Smith could well be prowling in other texts of hers. And the writings of these other authors might – like Emily Dickinson's – be found to contain hidden stories of trauma. The case of Stevens is especially likely, for he, like Kafka, spent his life working in accident insurance. Another possible avenue, in the case of the early twentieth century, would be to challenge our usual way of categorizing literature: as either modernist (Joyce, Proust, Kafka) or war literature (Sassoon, Barbusse, Jünger). Perhaps these works now need to be read together, within the same constellation of trauma and the same crisis of meaning – a crisis that is at once medical and literary.

Hoffmann at the Battle of Dresden: "The Sandman" and the Napoleonic Wars

E.T.A. Hoffmann was an eyewitness to the Napoleonic Wars – notably the wars' second largest battle, in August 1813, in the Saxon capital of Dresden. In this battle, the city suffered casualties totalling almost 60,000 and its worst bombardment till the Anglo-American attack of 1945 (figures 1–2). Hoffmann had arrived in Dresden in April, at the beginning of Napoleon's bloody German Campaign, when the city was already teeming with soldiers. Napoleon headquartered in Dresden intermittently during that spring and summer, and Hoffmann experienced the thrill of seeing "the Emperor" but also the stress of pre-battle tension. Hoffmann watched Napoleon and the Grande Armée enter the city on May 8, chasing the retreating Russians and Prussians. Skirmishes broke out. The Russians exploded the Elbe Bridge, and on the following day, Hoffmann witnessed a "continual bombardment" back and forth between French and Russian troops. Hoffmann and many other civilians were caught in the crossfire. He recorded in his diary that a volley of bullets ricocheted nearby and almost hit him (T 455).

The Grande Armée moved on, and in late August, with Napoleon off attacking the Silesians, the combined Russian, Prussian, and now Austrian forces surrounded the remaining French and Westphalian troops in Dresden. Hoffmann, like the other trapped civilians, worried for his safety. On August 22, he moved his family from their pleasant house in the suburbs to inside the city walls. Noting this "highly disquieting day" in his diary, he watched nervously as the Russians and Prussians approached. On August 23, he reports even "greater turmoil than yesterday." The cannon fire is getting closer. He sees bleeding French soldiers retreating to the city and even

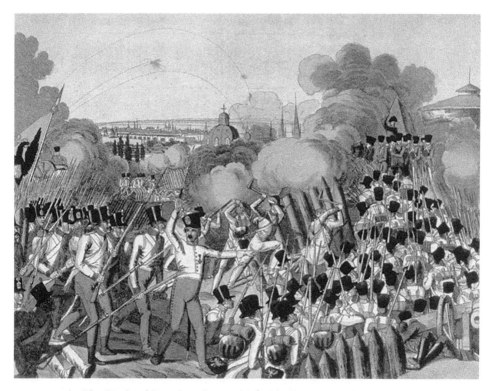

1. The Battle of Dresden, August 26–7, 1813. Artist unknown, ca. 1820

encounters a mutilated officer with "both eyes shot out." On August 24, the Russians are just outside the walls; Hoffmann hears "perpetual shooting." On August 25, the Russians and French skirmish before the city gates. A stream of "bloody and screaming" soldiers retreats into town, and falling bombs set fire to a house. But these are still just scuffles. As Hoffmann notes in the expansion of his diary that he planned to publish as a pamphlet for his friends, a "strong army" has now – on the evening of August 25 – ominously "encircled" Dresden (T 469, Dv 803–4).

The "thunder of cannons" wakes Hoffmann on the next day, August 26. Later that morning, he sees Napoleon on horseback – having returned in an attempt to save the city. By the afternoon, Hoffmann realizes that an allied force of over 200,000 men has

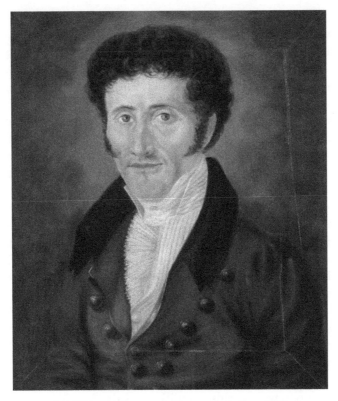

2. E.T.A. Hoffmann. Self-portrait, before 1822

begun a massive bombardment. The earth "quaked" beneath his feet and the windows "trembled" (*zitterten*). Shells landed all around, destroying even the house right across from him. After every explosion, he hears the "cries of woe" of the injured. And he is almost killed himself. A grenade flies "whizzing and crackling over my head," landing just ten steps from him. He later sees the fate that was nearly his. A similar shell lands nearby, hitting a soldier and shattering his head. Another bomb hits a civilian, tearing open his body till "his intestines fall out." Hoffmann pronounces this "one of the most remarkable days of my life" (T 469–70, Dv 804–6).

The next day, Napoleon drives the enemy into retreat – his last-ever victory – and peace returns to the city. Two days later, on

August 29, the shaken but curious Hoffmann decides to visit the main battlefield just outside the city. Thousands of soldiers lie already dead, and thousands more are alive but maimed, left on the field to die. The French lie naked in hastily dug pits with twenty or thirty bodies apiece. The whole field is covered with Russians, "mutilated and torn asunder [*zerrissen*] in the most horrible way." Hoffmann sees everywhere gruesomely disfigured bodies: "corpses with shattered heads [*zerschmetterten Köpfen*] and torsos"; one with "half of his head torn off"; and an officer frozen in fighting stance, holding high his sabre in his right hand, with his left arm ripped off and his breast shattered. At the end Hoffmann comes across a living casualty, a man whose feet have been "shot to pieces in the most pathetic way, such that everything stuck together with clotted blood." These images remind Hoffmann of his own inner life. As he tells us emphatically, he sees here the realization of his private fantastical visions: "What I have so often seen in dreams has come true – in a dreadful way – mutilated disjointed [*zerrissene*] humans!!" (Dv 808, T 471).

What role does this "remarkable day," in which Hoffmann's nightmares "come true," play in his life and art? At first glance, the role seems to be minimal. Hoffmann kept his normal diary during the battle and started expanding portions of it into a pamphlet entitled "Three Fateful Months!" ("Drei verhängnisvolle Monate!"). But he stopped writing this pamphlet one day in mid-sentence and never finished. He then described parts of the battle's aftermath in a leaflet, "The Vision on the Battlefield near Dresden" ("Die Vision auf dem Schlachtfelde bei Dresden," 1814), but even here he quickly detoured from the actual battle to an allegorical vision of the "tyrant" (Napoleon) as a daemon of myth. "The Poet and the Composer" (1813) similarly begins with a realistic account of Dresden – the bombardment of an unnamed "city" – but then shifts to a dialogue about the respective merits of poetry and music. In Hoffmann's three later works that explicitly mention the Napoleonic Wars, Dresden is dropped completely: "The Dei of Elba in Paris" (1815) describes Napoleon's Hundred Days before Waterloo, "The Uncanny Guest" (1818) transports us back to the anti-Napoleonic uprisings in Spain, and "The Elementary Spirit" (1821) narrates a Prussian officer's return home after the wars have ended.

It is as if Hoffmann has achieved the goal that he set for himself in the midst of his tense wartime stay in Dresden. He would use fiction as an escape, he said in August 1813, to turn away from the actual tragedy he was witnessing:

> Never has writing so appealed to me as in this dark and fateful time, when one ekes out one's existence and is happy to have it – It is as if I have unlocked for myself a wondrous kingdom, a kingdom that emerges from within me and, as it takes shape, transports me away from pressures of external events [*des Äußern*]. (SW 1:301)

Hoffmann indeed sat down shortly after the bombing of Dresden and invented a wondrous kingdom. Although he had had this kingdom in mind for a while, he then, in the post-battle fall of 1813, put it on paper. The subtitle of this bestselling work, *The Golden Pot: A Modern Fairy Tale*, explicitly placed this realm far from "external events." Although the fairy tale's setting is nominally Dresden, the city of Hoffmann's trauma, this city bears no marks of the carnage he has seen. The war is completely erased. In the immediately subsequent years, Hoffmann continued this process of expurgation, venturing ever further into the world of fantasy, publishing *Fantasy Pieces* (1814/15), which included *The Golden Pot*; *The Devil's Elixir* (1815); and *Night Pieces* (1816/17).

But does Hoffmann's Dresden tragedy really just vanish, as he had hoped and as most critics believe, into the "wondrous kingdom" of fantasy?[1] As I argue in this chapter, it reappears, in hidden form, where we would least expect it: in Hoffmann's most well-known story, one supposedly anchored in personal psychology and alchemical mysticism, "The Sandman" (written in 1815 and published in *Night Pieces*). The fact that no readers – including Freud, in his famous interpretation from *The Uncanny* – have noticed "The Sandman's" repetition of Hoffmann's Dresden experience speaks to the force with which Hoffmann represses it.[2] I do not wish to diminish the importance of the hero Nathanael's infantile traumas, as described by Freud, but I do want to claim that these anxieties are too obvious to produce the story's full "uncanny" effect, a sensation perceived by readers before and after Freud. A second, authorial, trauma – one that has remained obscured for over two hundred years – produces that uncanny thing which, in Schelling's words, "ought to have remained secret, hidden, latent, but has come to light."[3] And, as with most uncanny events, this one hides in plain sight: at the heart of Hoffmann's most celebrated story.

By unveiling this secret discourse of war behind "The Sandman," I aim both to provide a new reading of the story and to disclose its exemplarity for uncanniness itself – specifically as a descriptor of modern violence. Before Hoffmann's era, the word "uncanny" (*unheimlich*) was rarely used, and certainly not in its contemporary psychological sense.[4] Furthermore, no philosophical concept of the uncanny existed.[5] The late eighteenth century indeed "invented" the uncanny, but not, as Terry Castle insists, because of the philosophical clash between enlightened reason and vestigial animism.[6] Rather, as Anthony Vidler contends, the uncanny becomes a popular term because of a more common experience: the dislodging of people's general sense of "home" (*Heim*).[7] Around 1800, industrialization and modern warfare produced a widespread and "un-homely" (*un-heimlich*) alienation. Multitudes of rural inhabitants moved to the cities to work in factories, and the new weaponry of the Napoleonic Wars shocked, traumatized, and displaced tens of thousands of civilians – including Hoffmann. As Tolstoy wrote, these wars produced "the fundamental and essential" experience of modernity: mass migration in what seemed to be random directions, a zero-sum "movement of the mass of European peoples from west to east and afterwards from east to west."[8]

The result was a thoroughgoing feeling of uprootedness, exile, and homelessness, both literal and psychological. The seeds for the *un-heimlich* were sown. And the war story hidden in "The Sandman" opens up this uncanny scene. What Freud assumed was a personal trauma turns out also to be a social one, and this has its source in modernity's new forms of violence. Modern warfare creates unheard of shocks and displacements. When the effects of these are repressed, they return with the force of strangeness. The great uncanny power of "The Sandman" issues thus not only from Nathanael's childhood trauma but also from the return – at the levels of narratorial and authorial perspective – of this repressed shock of war.

Readers have long perceived that "The Sandman's" Nathanael is suffering from some sort of trauma.[9] As a young university student,

Nathanael falls into "utter melancholy" for an apparently trivial reason: a barometer salesman arrives at his door trying to make a deal. Nathanael realizes that this scene alone cannot be the cause of his profound malaise: "Only some quite private association rooted deep in my life could bestow such significance upon this event." With this in mind, he submits himself to something resembling psychoanalysis. Nathanael writes a letter to his friend Lothar but "mistakenly" mails it to Lothar's sister Clara (also Nathanael's fiancée); in this letter, Nathanael promises to report "quietly and patiently as much of my early youth as will suffice to make everything clear, distinct and vivid" (S 86). With Clara now serving as his therapist, Nathanael reveals a distressing event from his childhood that promises to explain his melancholia. As a boy, he had equated a friend of his father's, Coppelius, with the fairy-tale figure of the Sandman, who plucked out children's eyes. Coppelius visits Nathanael's father in the evenings to engage in alchemical experiments, and one night, these result in a powerful explosion that kills the father.

Coppelius disappears without a trace – until, decades later, this barometer salesman materializes. Nathanael now sees in this salesman, who calls himself Coppola, the reappearance of the "Sandman": Coppelius. Coppola thus embodies the repressed traumatic event that, according to Freud, returns later in life to engender "uncanny" psychic crises. Lurking behind this fictional calamity is an autobiographical one: Hoffmann's own father had abandoned the family when Hoffmann was three years old, and Hoffmann suffered from this shock his entire life (U 232n1).[10]

Although the importance of Hoffmann's paternal loss is undeniable, a careful reading of this scene from Nathanael's childhood – the blast that kills his father – reveals a second, more recent trauma in Hoffmann's life. What is this blast, which both Nathanael and Freud call an "explosion" (*Explosion*) (U 228, Ug 240; S 94, Sg 19)? What kind of explosion is it? In his initial description to Clara, Nathanael describes being torn from sleep in the middle of the night:

> There came a fearful detonation, like the firing of a cannon. The whole house rumbled; there was a clattering and rushing past the door of my room; the housedoor slammed with a crash … I cried in terror, and

leaped from the bed. Then I heard a piercing, despairing cry of woe and I rushed out to my father's room: the doors stood open, billows of choking smoke welled out towards me, the serving-maid was crying ... Before the billowing hearth, his face blackened with smoke and hideously distorted, my father lay dead on the floor, my sisters lamenting and wailing all around him, my mother unconscious beside him.

Nathanael is awoken by nothing other than a war scene: a cannon blast followed by wails, laments, and piercing cries. He then stumbles through thick smoke to find a mutilated corpse. The experience leaves Nathanael, not surprisingly, tormented for the remainder of the story and of his life: This "most dreadful moment ... has suspended a veil of gloom over my life" (S 93, 92).

This warlike trauma sheds light also on how Hoffmann describes Nathanael's earlier encounter with the Sandman/Coppelius. While spying on his father and Coppelius, Nathanael similarly sees "thick black smoke" rising, and suddenly everywhere around him appear human faces "without eyes – instead of eyes there were hideous black cavities." Stricken by a "wild terror," Nathanael screams and flees his "*Versteck*": his "hiding-place" or, in the military meaning that was primary in Hoffmann's day, his "cover" or "ambush." He is violently seized by Coppelius (S 91, Sg 17).

Although I do not aim to diagnose Nathanael, who has not been in a war, as a victim of war trauma, I do want to emphasize how Hoffmann's description of cannon fire, military cover, cries of woe, choking smoke, and distorted faces on corpses recalls his own war – the Battle of Dresden – from two years earlier. We see the explicit connection when examining closely the three above-mentioned texts that Hoffmann wrote during or immediately after the battle: his diary, his aborted expansion of portions of it ("Three Fateful Months!"), and "The Vision on the Battlefield Near Dresden." All three prefigure, often verbatim, Nathanael's experience. But Hoffmann scholars have somehow failed to notice this.

This oversight is remarkable when one considers, first, the word-for-word evidence. Before the violence begins, both Hoffmann (in Dresden) and Nathanael (in his bedroom) feel anticipatory "anguish" (restlessness, *Unruhe*). Both are woken from sleep by the blast of a "cannon" (*Geschütz*). Both then hear everywhere "cries of woe" (*Jammer*) and "lamenting and wailing" (*heulten und winselten*). Both rush through the "billowing" (*dampfende*) smoke of these post-"explosion" (*Explosion*) ruins, and they find "hideously" (*gräßlich*) damaged bodies. These exact same words appear in both the war reports and "The Sandman" (T 469, Dv 803–6, V 479–81, Sg 19).

Even when Hoffmann does not transfer his war language verbatim to "The Sandman," he conveys equivalent images. The explosions cause Hoffmann's house to "quake" and "tremble," and Nathanael's to "rumble." Hoffmann finds men "mutilated and disjointed [torn asunder, *zerrissen*] in the most horrific way," and Nathanael discovers his father "hideously distorted." Hoffmann then returns to a verbatim correspondence between war and fiction in the story's most important image: Nathanael's nightmarish vision of enucleation. Nathanael sees black "cavities" (*Höhlen*) where eyes should be. Hoffmann likewise encountered in the battle an officer with his "eyes shot out" and, on top of this, corpses with gaping "eye cavities" (*Augenhöhlen*) (Dv 804, 808, 803; V 479; Sg 19, 17).

Hoffmann furthermore experiences in Dresden a precursor of post-traumatic stress disorder that prefigures Nathanael's own: the Napoleonic-era "wind-of-the-cannonball" (*vent du boulet*) syndrome that left soldiers with mysterious anxieties and phobias when shells passed nearby without actually touching them. The theory was that the cannonball's "wind" actually caused physical disturbances in the inner ear.[11] Hoffmann senses something similar when the grenade flew "whizzing and crackling" just over his head – miraculously not injuring him physically but, as the battle continues, killing several others before his eyes (Dv 805). Nathanael likewise hears and feels the massive, frightening explosion in his house; it kills his father, yet he is not injured himself. Hoffmann and Nathanael both remain physically unscathed but have psychological symptoms: they are extremely "anxious" (*ängstlich*) – again, Hoffmann uses the same word – and worry, as Hoffmann does during the battle, about the future: "what will happen next!"[12] Just as this "explosion" marks one of the "most remarkable days of my life" for Hoffmann, the "explosion" produces for Nathanael the "most dreadful moment of my childhood."

Even though Nathanael has not been in a war, he displays these symptoms of the *vent du boulet* syndrome, and so appears as the romantic precursor of the great literary-realist trauma victims of the Napoleonic Wars: Fabrice del Dongo in Waterloo (*The Charterhouse of Parma*, 1839) and, from *War and Peace* (1867), Nikolai Rostov in Schöngrabern and Austerlitz, and Pierre Bezukhov in Borodino.[13] Fabrice, Nikolai, and Pierre, like Nathanael, suffer only minor injuries yet they must, as Pierre reports, endure hours of cannonballs "crackling and whistling" past them. This ultimately leaves them, like Nathanael, mentally unstable. In the case of Pierre, his future wife, Natasha, tells him after the battle that he somehow seems afflicted – even though he is physically uninjured. And this affliction is so mysterious that she can describe it only through a drift into ellipsis: "You are not like yourself ..." Most important, Pierre's symptoms – like those of Nathanael and, as I will discuss in chapter 3, Gregor Samsa – emerge only long after the fact. Tolstoy prefigures Freud's theory that traumatic symptoms appear only after a "latency" period, as something "deferred" (*nachträglich*): "As generally happens, Pierre only felt the full effects of the physical privation and strain he had suffered ... after they were over." He falls ill for three months with a mysterious ailment that confused the doctors, who resorted, Tolstoy tells us, to the catch-all diagnosis of "bilious fever."[14]

Nathanael develops similar symptoms of war trauma: psychic injuries without clear physical sources. Like other war veterans throughout modernity, including those treated by Freud's pupil Wilhelm Stekel in World War I (see my next chapter), Nathanael emerges from this cannon-like explosion unable to have romantic relations with his fiancée. What is more, he develops a hysterical belief that parts of his body have been amputated: the Sandman has "unscrewed my hands and feet," Nathanael shouts. He then has a "sudden spasm," feels "nothing more," and falls unconscious. He awakens long afterwards, "as if from the sleep of death." Here and for the rest of the story, Nathanael becomes a bundle of nervous energy, resembling not only veterans such as Tolstoy's Pierre from the Napoleonic Wars but also the war-shakers (*Kriegszitterer*) from the Great War one hundred years later. A "sudden spasm shot through my frame ['twitched through my nerves and bones,' *durchzuckte Nerv und Gebein*]." Later, "a spasm shuddered through him ['his pulse and veins twitched spasmodically,' *da zuckte es krampfhaft in seinen Pulsen und Adern*]," and he begins "raving and leaping high into the air." Right before he commits suicide, Nathanael screams twice, "*Feuerkreis*" – a word marked by Hoffmann in italics. Generally translated as "circle of fire!," *Feuerkreis* also means, in the nineteenth-century military parlance that Hoffmann knew firsthand from the armed "encircling" of Dresden, "*circle of gunfire!*" (S 92, 123, 124; Sg 18, 48, 49).

These correspondences reveal the semantic and thematic connections between "The Sandman" and the Battle of Dresden, but they do not explain everything – particularly not "The Sandman's" famously complicated use of point of view and the peculiar status of its narrator. The story seems in fact to begin without a narrator (with letters) until, roughly one-third of the way through, a narrator announces himself as a "friend" of Nathanael and his family, and as the holder of these letters (S 99, 101). A couple of pages later, the narrator fades into the background, telling the story mostly from Nathanael's perspective. On the final page, the narrator returns abruptly to offer his opinions on the tale. As if to alert his readers to the importance of perspective in the story, Hoffmann has Nathanael purchase a *Perspektiv* (meaning both "telescope" and "perspective") from Coppola. Nathanael uses this – specifically, a "Taschenperspektiv" (pocket telescope) – to observe his new beloved, Olimpia. And he looks through this same *Taschenperspektiv* – referred to ambiguously as "Coppola's *Perspektiv*" – just before he tries to kill Clara at the end. *Perspektiv*, in both of its senses, seems to offer the key to understanding the story's most important moments of love and violence. Why is Nathanael looking through a *Perspektiv* in these crucial scenes? And why is he looking through the *Perspektiv* of someone else ("Coppola's *Perspektiv*")? How might this confusion of perspective relate, if at all, to Hoffmann's experiences in the Battle of Dresden?

Hoffmann, it turns out, uses this same word – *Taschenperspektiv* – to describe what he sees at 11:00 on the morning of the great bombardment on August 26, 1813. Napoleon is standing on a bridge "looking frequently through a small *Taschenperspektiv* down the Elbe." What Nathanael later needs for erotic fantasy (to ogle Olimpia),

Napoleon now requires for war (to observe the enemy). Beyond this, we learn that Hoffmann himself has been using "a very good telescope" throughout the battle, probably also now to look at Napoleon. One man looks through a telescope and sees another man looking through a telescope. In a premonition of "The Sandman's" description of Nathanael looking through Coppola's *Perspektiv*, we see here the pressing question of both the war and the story: Whose *Perspektiv* is it?

Napoleon requires a good *Perspektiv* in Dresden to win the battle, but Hoffmann requires one for a different reason: to be a successful artist. Only because of his "very good telescope" can Hoffmann see clearly the drama unfolding before him: "the Emperor" with his own telescope consulting among his adjutants, the advance of "very strong Russian and Austrian columns," and, finally, the Prussians storming the trenches at the city walls (Dv 804). To heighten this perspective, Hoffmann spends the first part of the day in the attic of a neighbouring apartment building, which he calls his "observatory." But when shells destroy the roofs of nearby buildings, Hoffmann realizes that his observatory is unsafe. He heads down the stairs and on to the street. But he is even more exposed here; this is where the shell nearly kills him. He proceeds to his own building and hides there with others in a staircase – deliberately "away from the window," surrendering vision for survival. Bombs fall everywhere, landing even in the alley right behind him. After each explosion, Hoffmann hears horrible "cries of woe." Surmising that a battery of guns has been aimed at his neighbourhood, he sneaks out the back and runs to the home of a friend, Keller.

From Keller's building, Hoffmann regains his vantage point and observes the entire catastrophe: the smashed skull of the soldier, the ripped-open intestines of the civilian, and the horrible injuries of three others in front of the Frauenkirche. Hoffmann drinks a glass of wine with Keller and proclaims an aesthetics of terror: "What is life! Not being able to bear the touch of a red-hot iron, how weak is human nature!" While Keller is frightened by the continued bombing, Hoffmann keeps his cool and his artist's perspective. Keller "ließ sein Glas fallen" – meaning either "let his glass [of wine] drop" or, as in the archaic English usage of "glass," "let his glass [telescope] drop." The pun is, for Hoffmann, clear. Although Hoffmann had called Napoleon's telescope a *Perspektiv*, he now calls his own a *Glas*. When Keller lets his *Glas* drop and Hoffmann does not, Hoffmann drives home the double entendre: the sovereignly cool narrator of a brutal scene can drop neither his wine nor his telescope. Like the objective bird's-eye narrator of nineteenth-century realism, Hoffmann must remain unruffled: "God preserve my calm [*Ruhe*] and courage while in mortal danger" (Dv 806).

Only from this posture of detachment can he observe the full extent of the violence. He now reports dramatically, underlining his words, of a chambermaid being "*torn asunder* [*zerrissen*] in the strictest sense of the word." He then watches as a midwife peeks out of her window and has "her head ripped off." A clerk, minding his own business in his office, loses an arm (Dv 807). On this most remarkable day, Hoffmann moves from being within the fray – a "character" nearly killed by a shell while in the street – to being above it. Both survival and artistic vision, he learns, are matters of *Perspektiv*.

In "The Sandman," we see a similar tension between proximity and distance, specifically in the narrator, who resembles that other narrator: Hoffmann, the reporter at the Battle of Dresden. At the moment when "The Sandman's" narrator announces himself in the story, he does so as a *character*, someone on the stage along with the others. He has a recognizable personality: energetic, loquacious, and excitable. What is more, he is a friend of Nathanael, Clara, and Lothar, and seems close to the entire family (Lothar and Clara are Nathanael's stepsiblings). This is why Lothar entrusts him with the letters.

Yet this intimacy also explains what appears to be an important difference between this narrator and Hoffmann in Dresden. Whereas Hoffmann remains calm during the massacre in Dresden, the narrator is devastated by what has happened to his "poor friend," Nathanael. He is unable to speak or write. His speech "dissolve[s]" into non-linguistic "sighing"; he can only "stammer and stutter." His friends ask him "What is wrong?" but he cannot say. It is as if the traumatic event has *happened to him*. He indeed asks his readers: have you ever felt the need "to compress everything marvellous, glorious, terrible, joyful, harrowing that had *happened to you* into the very first word" (my emphasis)? This trauma of witnessing, which has "happened to" the narrator, leaves him with symptoms similar to those of Nathanael. The narrator, too, is initially unable to speak of his distress: "every word ... seemed colourless and cold and dead." Only later, when the pain that he "bear[s] within" begins to overflow, do words appear. He is now, like Nathanael, overcome by the "strong compulsion" to speak (S 99–100).

This is when the narrator tells the second half of Nathanael's story, mostly from the point of view of this poor friend, with whom he now identifies. The narrator thus performs the experiment that Hoffmann had suggested when looking through his telescope at Napoleon looking through *his* telescope. What might it mean to adopt someone else's *Perspektiv*, especially during a traumatic moment? Can we sense what is happening to that other person? Is it possible to feel the ordeal as if it were "happening to you?" Hoffmann attempts this only twice, briefly, in his battle description. He imagines what is going through the mind of the civilian who has just been hit by a shell in his midsection. This man does not realize how hurt he is, Hoffmann guesses, which is why he is trying to "pull himself together" and act like nothing is wrong. But then this man sees his intestines spill out and realizes the truth. Hoffmann likewise witnesses Napoleon tossing his head "fiercely" back and forth, then imagines Napoleon's inner life and thoughts about the battle. Hoffmann intuits "a certain essence in [the Emperor] that I had never before perceived." In "The Sandman," the narrator conducts Hoffmann's war experiment more thoroughly. Although this narrator sometimes steps back for ironic commentary – as Hoffmann does in his observatory with his telescope and wine – he generally immerses himself, in this second half of the story, in the perspective of the traumatized character.

At key moments in Nathanael's story, the narrator even shifts into the more focused third-person perspective of free indirect speech – still a new, experimental style in Hoffmann's day.[15] In this form of narration, the narratorial and figural perspectives merge almost completely. As if to draw attention to this merging, Hoffmann shifts to this style at the precise moment when Nathanael looks through Coppola's *Perspektiv*. Nathanael "took out Coppola's glass ... and looked at [Olimpia]," and then he imagines dancing with her, exclaiming without attribution or quotation, in the hall-mark of free indirect style: "Ah!," "To dance with her! – with her!," and "But how to raise the courage to ask her, the queen of the fes-tivities, to dance? And yet!" (S 113, Sg 38–9).[16] The narrator seems to have surrendered fully his ironic distance. He now sees the world through Nathanael's eyes, just as Nathanael adopts, at the same time, Coppola's *Perspektiv*. Perspectives blur, and the enchanting Olimpia overwhelms momentarily both Nathanael and the narra-tor. This passion, like the earlier trauma, seems to be "happening to" both of them.

The narrator's displacement of himself onto Nathanael carries with it more risks than he, as Nathanael's "friend," had initially im-agined. Seeing the world through Nathanael's eyes does not merely mean identifying with him. Because Nathanael is looking through the *Perspektiv* of Coppola, the narrator has thrown himself into a *mise en abyme* of affinities. His perspective merges with his friend's, whose perspective has merged with the "evil" Coppelius's, symbol-izing also Nathanael's own monstrous narcissism. Shortly after this scene, the authorities deliver Nathanael to a madhouse, and the narrator, perhaps unsettled by his proximity to this madness, reas-serts his ironic distance.

After Nathanael's apparent cure, the narrator again surrenders this distance – also at a crucial moment. Clara and Nathanael, now apparently happy, climb the tower on the marketplace of their hometown. After reaching the top, Clara notices a bush below that seems to be moving. Nathanael reaches into his pocket and pulls out, again, "Coppola's telescope [*Perspektiv*]." The deranging capac-ity of this perspective becomes immediately clear. Instead of looking down (at the bush), Nathanael looks, for no clear reason, "*seitwärts*" – sideways – a detail that is omitted from the standard English trans-lation (Sg 48, S 123). Nathanael's sideways perspective symbolizes the radical dislodging of his point of view into that of *someone else*. At precisely this point, the narrator again merges his perspective with Nathanael's through the unattributed exclamation of free indirect style: "Clara was standing before the glass!" Again, the narratorial and figural standpoints seem to become one – proclaiming a psy-chological situation that, as Samuel Weber points out, corresponds to the grammar of psychoanalysis.[17] Hoffmann's free indirect style blurs the distinction between the narratorial first person ("I," *Ich*) and the figural third person ("he," *Er*) in a way that mirrors psychoanalysis. For Freud, using the vernacular pronoun "I" (*Ich*), insisted that our first-person "ego" can never fully separate itself from our third-person "id" (Freud uses "it" [*Es*]).

And psychoanalysis says more than this. The first person must deliberately traffic with the third person, Freud argues, in order for the *Ich* to fulfil its potential: "Wo Es war, soll Ich werden" (where *It/id* was, there *I/ego* shall come to be) (GW 15:86). But this adventure of the *Ich* into the territory of the *Es* does not necessarily have a happy ending. The *Ich* might indeed attain a heroic individuation, but part of this *Ich* could remain stuck here, traumatically immobilized at the site of unbearable truth – "where *Es* was."[18] This problem is writ large in this scene from "The Sandman." The narrator's first person displaces itself into the third person of the character, Nathanael. But this "he" is more complex than "I" had ever imagined. Through "his" (Nathanael's) desire for the perfect feminine object for the satisfaction of his narcissism, he has become as ghastly as the "evil" Coppelius. Nathanael's "he" has become the "it" of the amoral unconscious. When the narrator identifies with "him," the narrator's "I," now resembling the "he" of Nathanael, enters this territory where "it" was – and still is. The narrator's ego will not return unscathed.

How does this story of the narrator losing his "I" in a devastating "it" (Nathanael's tragic life) relate to Hoffmann's having his "I" embroiled, two years earlier, in the overwhelming "it" of the Battle of Dresden? Near the end of "The Sandman" and of Hoffmann's account of the battle, both of the "narrators" witness violent scenes that are tellingly similar. Hoffmann sees "corpses with shattered heads [*mit zerschmetterten Köpfen*]" and other "shattered heads" (*zerschmetterte Köpfe*) on the battlefield (T 471). Before this, he witnesses from Keller's building the brutal death of a soldier: "A grenade fell in the middle of the marketplace [*Markt*] and exploded – in that same moment a Westphalian soldier, who was about to get water from the pump, fell dead with his head shattered [*mit zerschmettertem Kopf*]" (Dv 806). The narrator from "The Sandman" observes likewise the gory incident beneath the tower after Lothar rescues Clara from Nathanael. Nathanael leaps from the tower onto the middle of the "marketplace" (*Markt*) and lies there "with his head shattered" (*mit zerschmettertem Kopf*) (S 124, Sg 49). The two "I"s, Hoffmann, and the narrator of "The Sandman," encounter an uncannily similar "it." Both see, as eyewitnesses, the same shocking, public violence: a *zerschmettertem Kopf* in the middle of the *Markt.*

And these two narrators react in remarkably similar ways. Hoffmann finishes his glass of wine while priding himself on maintaining his calm (*Ruhe*). The narrator, despite his earlier emotional identification with his "friend," now takes on an oddly cool distance – in "The Sandman's" famously perplexing final paragraph. Immediately after describing Nathanael's shattered head, the narrator reports nonchalantly of the tale's aftermath:

> Several years later, you could have seen Clara, in a distant part of the country, sitting with an affectionate man hand in hand before the door of a lovely country house and with two lovely children playing at her feet, from which it could be concluded that Clara found in the end that quiet [*ruhige*] domestic happiness which was so agreeable to her cheerful disposition and which the inwardly riven [*zerrissene*] Nathanael could never have given her. (S 125, Sg 50)

Readers have generally viewed this ending either as a condemnation of Nathanael's narcissism[19] or as the narrator's ironic criticism of Clara's cold rationality. The second approach poses a vital question: After living so long with an apparently mentally ill fiancé, being nearly murdered by him, and then watching him commit suicide, how could Clara simply distance herself from all of this and live in "quiet domestic happiness"? Would this not require, the critics ask, a massive dose of callousness, self-delusion, and repression?[20]

Even though these two interpretations take opposite positions regarding whether Nathanael or Clara is to blame, they share one thing: a conflation of the narrator with Hoffmann. Whether focusing on Nathanael's romantic narcissism or Clara's cold practicality, both readings forget that the speaker at the end of the story is not a disinterested author making impartial moral judgments, but a narrator who, as a character in the story, has stakes in how we interpret it. And even if the critics do acknowledge that this voice is the narrator's – and thus subjective – they do not consider that the author's perspective, Hoffmann's, might be completely opposed to the narrator's. Both approaches thus overlook the story's most pressing question, which is the same question that we normally ask about Clara but that we must now ask about the narrator: After living so long with a mentally ill friend, sharing his emotional perspective, and then watching him commit suicide, how could *the narrator* possibly seem so unaffected by this story? Without, that is, a massive dose of callousness, self-delusion, and repression?

To answer this, let us return to the moment of Nathanael's violent death and ask whether we can locate the narrator physically, as a character in the story. We cannot know for certain, but details suggest that he could well have been present – as Hoffmann was in Dresden when the soldier died in front of him. The narrator is a friend of the family, perhaps growing up in the same hometown and in any case intimately enough related to be the recipient of the family's horrifying private letters. Earlier on the day of Nathanael's death, after Nathanael awoke from a deep sleep caused by his first nervous breakdown, the narrator tells us that Nathanael's friends and family were gathered round. Was the narrator too? If yes, did he take the fateful walk with the group to the marketplace?

The story's perspective suggests as much. The narrator reports on the many people, including Coppelius, who gathered at the foot of the tower while Nathanael raged at the top:

> Some wanted to enter the tower and overpower the madman [Nathanael], but Coppelius laughed and said: "Don't bother: he will soon come down by himself," and gazed upward with the rest. Nathanael suddenly stopped as if frozen; then he stooped, recognized Coppelius, and with the piercing cry: "Ha! Lov-ely *occe!* Lov-ely *occe!*" he jumped over the parapet.
> As Nathanael was lying on the pavement with his head shattered [*mit einem zerschmettertem Kopf*], Coppelius disappeared into the crowd. –

In this description, Coppelius speaks at normal volume: "Don't bother." There is no exclamation point, no shouting. In order to hear this, the narrator must have been standing near Coppelius, in the same crowd. The narrator furthermore seems to share the group's visual perspective from below. He watches as Nathanael stands frozen, then "stoop[s]" down to peer at Coppelius, then leaps over the parapet to land at the feet of the crowd (S 124, Sg 49).

If the narrator is indeed among this throng, we now have an explanation for what he earlier called *his own* trauma – for what made it so difficult for him to tell the story in the first place. He was suffering for years from a horrifying pain "within." This rendered him speechless and made all words seem "cold and dead." And we can understand why: he had been standing in the marketplace of his hometown among a group of neighbours when his "poor friend" sprang to his death (S 99).

The narrator's detachment in this final paragraph now takes on the full meaning of repression, and "The Sandman" reveals itself as a traumatic narrative. The dash that appears after Nathanael's death, missing from the English translation, marks the repression of this trauma: "As Nathanael was lying on the pavement with his head shattered, Coppelius disappeared into the crowd. –" The sorrow of the mourning narrator, the witness to the friend's trauma, hangs on this dash. Only after the temporal break signified typographically by this *Gedankenstrich* ("stroke of thought"), can the narrator's words return. A paragraph break follows, as well as a passage of "years." Then the narrator can finally speak, but he is unable to see the truth remaining locked in the dash. He releases instead his false story of repression.

This repression returns us to the Battle of Dresden. Is it really possible that Hoffmann, the battle's narrator, watched the massacre at his feet with such coldness – as he records in the aborted expansion of his diary? After seeing the Westphalian soldier get his "head shattered" while pumping water, does Hoffmann really just keep "looking comfortably out the window" with a glass of wine in his hand? Does he really, after this bloody death, just "drain" this glass and bellow, "What is life! Not being able to bear the touch of a red-hot iron, how weak is human nature!"? If this indeed is how he reacts, is it false bravado? An attempt to protect himself from the fear caused by this "damned anxious" day (Dv 806)? Does Hoffmann, like the narrator of "The Sandman," actually "bear within" a great, deep pain from watching others die at close range? Does this explain why Hoffmann one day simply halts this reworking of his diary in mid-sentence?

In this reworking, which he had planned to publish as a pamphlet for his friends, Hoffmann describes these deaths in the city and then the devastation he sees on the battlefield while touring it three days later. He wades through disfigured corpses and stumbles across one living man whose feet are so mangled by shells that "everything stuck together with clotted blood." The man was begging for water. Hoffmann writes, "how good it was that I ..." Then he simply stops (Dv 808). A few months later, in a December 1813 letter to his friend Carl Friedrich Kunz, Hoffmann lies about the status of this expanded diary. He claims that he had completed the revised text and, by mistake (like Nathanael!), sent it to a different friend (SW 1:322). But the broken-off manuscript tells a different story.[21] Hoffmann cannot finish, and more than this, he hides his inability to finish. Does the truth of repression reveal itself in this lie? Was Hoffmann ashamed of not being able "to bear the touch of a red-hot iron"? If yes, does the buried pain he has witnessed work itself out elsewhere, two years later, in the story of the narrator from "The Sandman"?

One last clue suggests as much. The final remark that Hoffmann makes in his actual (unrevised) diary on that fateful day, August 26, is incomplete. It is parenthetical, and more than this, both the closing parenthesis and the final period are missing: "(Multiple citizens were injured or killed today by shells" [*sic*]. Hoffmann's account of the battle ends here, with this unclosed parenthesis, reminding us of the dash that cannot close the narrator's story of Nathanael. We are left with the typographical open-endedness of shock, fear, and fatigue. When Hoffmann picks up his diary later to revise portions into a pamphlet for friends, he attempts to continue this open thought – specifically by describing some of these "citizens." He recounts one especially moving case, which I mentioned briefly above:

The chambermaid of Countess Breza stepped out the door, before which stood a carriage that was supposed to bring the Countess to safety in a different district, but in precisely that moment she [the chambermaid] was, in the strictest sense of the word, *torn asunder* [*zerrissen*] by a shell. (Dv 807, Hoffmann's emphasis)

Hoffmann depicts the chambermaid as "zerrissen," just like the "mutilated disjointed [*zerrissene*] humans" he saw "torn asunder [*zerrissen*]" on the battlefield. And he will soon depict Nathanael in exactly this same way: as "zerrissen."

Hoffmann's narrator in the "The Sandman" indeed uses this adjective, now in its figurative sense, to describe his friend in the final phrase of the final sentence of the story: Nathanael, he says, was inwardly "riven" or "torn asunder" (*zerrissen*). Because Nathanael was so psychologically "zerrissen," he could never have made Clara happy. But the narrator knows that, just two sentences earlier, he had described another reason why Nathanael could never have made Clara happy: because he was dead, torn asunder "in the strictest sense of the word," just like the chambermaid. Nathanael's head had been smashed on the plaster.

This prefiguring of Nathanael's tearing asunder by the chambermaid's tearing asunder takes us beyond "The Sandman's" narrator and beyond the story itself: to Hoffmann witnessing that literal tearing asunder two years before writing the story. Hoffmann claimed not to have been traumatized – he just kept drinking his wine – but the reappearance of the chambermaid's torn body in Nathanael's torn body suggests otherwise. If Hoffmann, the war narrator, has indeed reconstituted part of himself in the fictional narrator of "The Sandman," then he has not done so in the cool, conscious way that critics claim. Hoffmann is not the romantic ironist criticizing Clara's heartless rationality. Rather, he is emotionally present in this narrator through his earlier witnessing of an unspeakable trauma. The historical trauma of Dresden is not obvious in the story. It is hidden, even from Hoffmann himself, yet it is precisely this cover-up that creates "The Sandman's" uncanny effect. The trauma is available to us only in veiled form. We see merely clues – the explosion, the shattered head, the tearing asunder – that point to that concealed thing that is always only beginning to come to light.

The fact that readers of "The Sandman" have not noticed this for two centuries returns us to the main theme of Hoffmann's story: The Sandman blinds us, puts dirt in our eyes, threatens even to pluck them out. Nathanael is terrified of losing his eyes, as we all are – for we fear the actual and figurative blindness emphasized by Freud and by post- and even anti-Freudian readers. As critics of Freud argue, the story's uncanniness issues not just from a fear of castration but also from the blindness produced by ever-shifting perspectives. These rob Nathanael – and Freud and us – of a view of the truth.[22] Yet even this insight into blindness has remained blind to the history of Hoffmann's own traumatic eyewitnessing. Hoffmann, the narrator of the Battle of Dresden, sees the importance of having a *Perspektiv* – a telescope and a perspective – when seeking the truth of historical violence. He even imagines looking through the "other" *Perspektiv* of Napoleon and of the battle's victims. When this leaves Hoffmann traumatized and metaphorically blinded himself, he attempts it again, however unconsciously, in "The Sandman." He loses himself in others' perspectives, as these others lose themselves in the perspectives and telescopes of yet others, and so on. In this way, Hoffmann provides us with a brilliant account of the blindness inherent even in attempts to overcome blindness, especially when we are attempting to see something traumatic.

My aim, in this chapter and this book, is not just to read "The Sandman" and other modern texts as traumatic narrations. I also want to make an exemplary argument about a certain type of modern writing. Readers often claim that this writing – known as "romanticism" or "modernism" – produces its uncanny effect through its metafictional relation to itself. Neil Hertz's classic essay about "The Sandman" is a case in point. For Hertz, the key to understanding the climactic scene – Nathanael leaping to his death – lies in the earlier appearance of the word that Nathanael eventually screams at the end: "Feuerkreis." Nathanael had included this word in a poem, which is, Hertz argues, the perfect example of metafiction or "romantic irony." For this poem has the same plot as "The Sandman" itself: Coppelius's destruction of Nathanael's "happiness" with Clara. For Hertz, the internal repetition of this word and this story is evidence against Freud's claim that the uncanny effect emerges primarily from childhood trauma, as experienced by both Nathanael and Hoffmann.[23]

Instead, Hertz continues, we must understand this story, and "The Sandman" itself, as being about no event in particular. Nathanael's desire to write a pure and perfect poem corresponds rather to the narrator's desire to create "living shapes" that will entrance readers. This corresponds in turn to Hoffmann's own "literary ambitions." What is unsettling is not Nathanael's trauma but the "illusion of infinite regress" that these texts within texts create. Writing's endless *mise en abyme* is upsetting because it refers only to itself, frighteningly suggesting that we cannot connect literature – or language in general – to our world. Language becomes terrifyingly non-referential, pointing only to itself, to its own "uncontrollable repetition," and to a world without meaning.[24]

Hertz's "literary" argument, repeated by subsequent deconstructivist readers,[25] challenges not only Freud's "traumatic" interpretation but also my own – unless, that is, we consider how this discourse of literary undecidability relates to the discourse of trauma itself. In the nineteenth century, victims of wars and of train accidents presented symptoms that did not connect clearly to injuries. Doctors originally supposed that these symptoms had physical causes: inner ear damage in the "wind-of-the-cannonball" syndrome from Hoffmann's day, damage to the spine from railway accidents in the late nineteenth century, and molecular disturbances to the brain during World War I. But this "pathological-anatomical substrate" remained "undetectable." The "submicroscopic" cause of suffering was the missing origin; molecular damage could not be proven. In this way, the "ultramodern" medical language of hermeneutic undetectability mirrored the language of literature's non-referentiality,[26] both in "The Sandman" and in the deconstructivist readings of the text.

We can now begin to see how this language contains a significance beyond semiotic self-reference or even the impossibility to signify. This opaqueness points instead to the medical language surrounding the traumatized body itself. The indecidability of the sign is also the unreadability of the symptomatic body. Such bodies haunt texts long interpreted as working against referentiality, including, as discussed in my introduction, those written a century after "The

Sandman": Joyce's *Ulysses*, Proust's *In Search of Lost Time*, and Mann's *The Magic Mountain*. These bodies trouble "The Sandman" and, uncannily, also the apparently ahistorical text that claimed to have solved "The Sandman's" mysteries: Freud's *The Uncanny* (1919). We see here, as I will demonstrate in the next chapter, a series of apparently traumatized bodies that recall the violence of Freud's own war that has just concluded. Yet Freud never mentions this connection. Because what turns out to be most uncanny is trauma itself. It is always present and absent, known and unknown, on the tips of our tongues yet never spoken. For Hoffmann it was the Napoleonic Wars. For Freud, it is the recurrence of these wars a century later, in 1914. War trauma is the secret of "The Sandman," which then becomes the secret of *The Uncanny*. The repressed always returns at least twice, and each time it becomes harder to name.

Chapter Two

Freud and World War I: The Uncanny Trauma of Contagion

We use the term "uncanny" to describe many things: a frightening film, a disturbing encounter, even a haunting act of violence such as the attacks of 9/11.[1] The term had indeed become so trendy already by the 1990s that Martin Jay ironically entitled an essay "The Uncanny Nineties." Yet despite our reliance on the term, we have little sense of what it means or where it comes from. It seems that its very slipperiness is what makes it indispensable: we need an indefinable concept to explain the inexplicable. Deconstructionist interpreters cemented this indefinability in the 1970s, on the heels of Jacques Derrida's momentous 1970 footnotes on Freud's *The Uncanny* in "La double séance." They consistently viewed uncanniness as an exemplary self-unravelling term that exposed the vacuum at the heart of all concept-making.[2]

Samuel Weber, one of the most insightful of these readers, saw a theoretical dead end in equating the uncanny with "indecidability" – insisting instead that we investigate the term's "historical status."[3] But this call went unheeded for decades. Scholars continued to assume that the uncanny, unlike other concepts, was somehow divorced from social, linguistic, and philosophical contexts. This supposition of ahistoricity is especially egregious for the uncanny because of its radical modernity. Unlike terms such as truth, beauty, and sublimity, the word uncanny (*unheimlich*) was rarely even used before 1800 and did not enter theoretical debates until a century later (see chapter 1). Only in 1992 did Anthony Vidler begin to address this modernity, claiming that the concept emerged out of the sense of un-homeliness and estrangement in late nineteenth- and early twentieth-century Europe. Vidler discussed the most significant contemporaneous essay on the topic – Freud's 1919 *The Uncanny* – and briefly noted its specific context: World War I and the "barbaric regression" of the European "homeland."[4]

Vidler's association of Freud's essay to World War I strikes us today as obvious. Although Freud did not complete *The Uncanny* until 1919, he wrote much of it during the hostilities, beginning even as early as 1913, and he mentions the war twice – once explicitly and once implicitly, as the "times in which we live" (U 244, 220). More than this, he composed the essay in the midst of his other attempts to grapple, directly or indirectly, with the war's effects: "Thoughts for the Times on War and Death" (1915), "On Transience" (1916), and "Mourning and Melancholia" (1917). Given these links, it is surprising only that scholars have taken so long to connect *The Uncanny* to the war. There is to this day only one monograph dedicated to Freud and World War I, from 1975, and it never mentions *The Uncanny* (Büttner, *Freud und der Erste Weltkrieg*). Even in the wake of Vidler, such associations remained cursory – with the war generally mentioned only as period atmosphere within larger arguments devoted to different aspects of the essay. Readers seem to have accepted Freud's claim that the war was primarily background noise: merely difficult "times" that prevented Freud from obtaining secondary literature – peripheral to an essay that is actually concerned with something else.[5]

But what if *The Uncanny*'s relation to the war is deeper and more essential? In the one paragraph Vidler devotes to the war, he speculates on how it might have influenced Freud's essay: "'The Uncanny' seems to incorporate, albeit in an unstated form, many observations on the nature of anxiety and shock that [Freud] was unable to include in the more clinical studies of shell shock."[6] Readers of the chronologically ordered *Standard Edition* realize that Freud published *The Uncanny* in the midst of texts devoted to shell shock (called "war neurosis" in Austria and Germany): his introduction to *Psycho-Analysis and the War Neuroses* (1919); his "Memorandum on the Electrical Treatment of War Neurotics" (1920); and *Beyond the Pleasure Principle*, which was inspired partially by "the war neuroses" issuing from "the terrible war which has just ended" (SE 18:12). Despite this context, Freud's observations on war and shock in *The Uncanny* have never been catalogued, perhaps because they are generally indirect.[7] But they are numerous enough to constitute a sustained collective unconscious.

Especially remarkable is Freud's recounting of a popular 1917 English story that describes a traumatized soldier returning home, which gives us a hint at why Freud's references to war and shock remain unstated. This tale turns out to be vital to Freud's central claim about the uncanny: that it results from the unexpected return of the repressed. For this story presents Freud with the most striking exemplar of such a return in postwar Europe: the traumatized soldier, given up for dead, coming back to haunt the home front – in the English story as well as in Freud's own wartime dreams. This soldier is present also in Freud's primary example of the uncanny, E.T.A. Hoffmann's "The Sandman," whose language refers back to the trauma that Hoffmann witnessed on a Napoleonic battlefield near Dresden in 1813.

The fact that Freud does not name this trauma in *The Uncanny* speaks only to the complexity of the problem it poses. In *The Uncanny*, I maintain, Freud begins to see phantasmagorical, psychosocial aspects to war shock that he could not address in his more clinical writings. His inability to state this directly even in *The Uncanny* creates a deeper uncanny effect within the essay itself. *The Uncanny* stages the same "return of the repressed" that it diagnoses. In this chapter, I aim first to delineate this staging and, later, to propose its conceptual relevance. The shadow of the war forces us to understand the Freudian "uncanny" differently: not just as a personal trauma but as a symptom of the social repression of this trauma. The real horror of the uncanny, Freud's essay teaches us, is not our own but *the other's trauma* – embodied in wartime Europe by the war neurotic and his apparently contagious affliction.

Freud first mentions the war through an apology, claiming that the "times in which we live" have made it difficult for him to acquire foreign literature, and by the end of the essay's second section, he implies more specifically the war's relation to trauma. After alluding twice to the war-inspired *Beyond the Pleasure Principle* (U 238, 242), he describes a particular event – the advertisements of clairvoyants in the streets of wartime Vienna:

> In our great cities, placards announce lectures that undertake to tell us how to get into touch with the souls of the departed; and it cannot be denied that not a few of the most able and penetrating minds among our

men of science have come to the conclusion ... that a contact of this kind
is not impossible. (U 242)

Freud does not need to mention the war for his 1919 readers to
know that these "departed" are the millions of young men who never
returned from the battlefields. Many of them disappeared in the mud
of the trenches, in unimaginable conditions, leaving behind relatives
attempting to contact them. Rudolf Steiner's Anthroposophical Society, the British Spiritualists' National Union, and the practice of
clairvoyance flourished in these years – with clairvoyants even being
outlawed in some warring countries.[8] The English soldier-poet Robert
Graves recalls a mother knocking on the wall of her missing son's bedroom throughout an entire night: "There were thousands of mothers
like her, getting in touch with their dead sons by various spiritualistic
means."[9] And the Australian artist Norman Lindsay remembers "that
universal sense of shocked insecurity due to the 1914 war which sent
nearly everybody into the back-parlour limbo of Spiritualism."[10]

The "penetrating minds" who believed in this included Freud's
beloved Arthur Conan Doyle, who used a "Red Indian spirit" to con-
verse with his dead soldier son,[11] and Thomas Mann, who attended
séances regularly beginning in 1919 and even added one to the plot of
The Magic Mountain.[12] The 1919 film *Nerven* (*Nerves*), which appeared
in German cinemas concurrently with *The Uncanny*, speaks to the
popular appeal of this belief. It begins with a mother telepathically
experiencing a breakdown together with her own son on the front.
Rhythmic cuts from the mother at home to the son in his trench make
it seem that the mother is suffering convulsions at the same time as
he is. A contemporaneous reviewer said that the film depicted an "epidemic of the nerves," an epidemic that apparently infected not just
the mother but even the film's viewers.[13] They reported suffering similar fits – until, that is, the authorities withdrew *Nerves* from cinemas.[14]

Freud discusses this belief in telepathy in the context of modern
man's "uncanny," vestigial belief in "the return of the dead." Even
today, Freud insists, we think we see "spirits and ghosts," fantasies
which have changed remarkably little since primeval times:

Since almost all of us still think as savages do [about death], it is no matter for surprise that the primitive fear of the dead is still so strong within

us and always ready to come to the surface on any provocation. Most likely our fear still implies the old belief that the dead man becomes the enemy of his survivor and seeks to carry him off to share his new life with him. (U 241–2)

This image of the dead man rising up to take revenge is of course ancient, but it would also have reminded Freud's readers of the present: of stories circulating about German soldiers stuck in craters with enemy corpses for days, a major cause of the soldiers' own "unheimlich" belief in ghosts.[15] Moreover, Freud's dead man transforming into the "enemy of his survivor" recalls Freud's earlier essay about the war, "Thoughts for the Times on War and Death," in which he explains that we fear our dead loved ones even more than we fear our dead enemies. For our love for our intimates was always shamefully ambivalent. When they die, as part of us had wished, we feel guilty. This guilt transforms our loved ones into revenge-seeking spectres: they become "evil demons" that are "to be dreaded" (SE 14:294). Although we eventually distort this dread into "an unambiguous feeling of piety," as Freud writes in *The Uncanny*, our fear never subsides (U 243). This would especially have been true following a war in which most of the surviving parents, like Freud, had uncritically sent their sons off to battle.

Just one page later, Freud alludes specifically to the trauma of these soldier sons, claiming that, for many people, the thought of "being buried alive … is the most uncanny thing of all" (U 244). Freud claims that this reminds us of our repressed "lascivious fantasy" of returning to the womb, but a premature burial would also have revived in Freud's readers a different image, specifically the predominant traumatic one from World War I: being buried alive in the trenches – as opposed to the main vision of trauma from World War II, "Blitzkrieg." Just one year later, Freud indeed refers to "being buried by a fall of earth" (*Erdverschüttung*) as one of the two main causes of trauma in World War I (SE 17:212, GW Nachtragsband: 707). Tens of thousands of soldiers died during the Great War in collapsed trenches, most notably in the June 7, 1917 Battle of Messines, where the British detonated 600 tons of explosives beneath the German lines. This caused the largest man-made explosion ever (until the first atomic bomb test), creating shock waves as far as

London.[16] The German trenches crumpled, killing 10,000 soldiers immediately and wounding tens of thousands more, many of whom returned home traumatized. This fear of being buried alive – being "verschüttet" – is a staple of war chronicles: Erich Maria Remarque finds comrades "verschüttet" in the foxhole next to his.[17] Ernst Jünger repeatedly fears "Verschüttung," and he, like Remarque, rushes to excavate a comrade who is "verschüttet" in a nearby hole.[18]

Freud's insights drew on those of Hermann Oppenheim, one of Germany's leading neurologists. Already in 1889, Oppenheim had identified "traumatic neurosis" as a distinct clinical disorder, claiming that violent commotions caused by railway accidents damaged the fine tissue of the brain and produced neurotic symptoms. This theory was controversial, as I will discuss in the following chapter, but it led to changes in the insurance industry and rendered railways liable, for the first time, for neurotic injury. During the war, Oppenheim led the wing for nervous illness at the reserve hospital in Berlin's Museum of Applied Arts; he later directed the Berlin Military Hospital for Nervous Diseases. Oppenheim met many "war shakers" (*Kriegszitterer*) and developed a theory that these men, like the survivors of railway collisions, were suffering from neuroses ("war neuroses"), which he considered to be a subset of the traumatic neuroses. The cause was not only the well-known explosion of shells but also – as Oppenheim argued in 1916, a few years ahead of Freud – "Verschüttung."[19]

Jünger's description during the battle of Guillemont that same year illustrates Oppenheim's point. A British shell buries alive ("verschüttet") a man in a nearby foxhole. When Jünger and his comrades excavate him, they find him alive yet half-dead: "exhausted to death," with his face "sunken in, like a skull and bones" (see figure 3).[20] The man is never the same, instilled now with a mad fear of being buried. During the next shelling, his comrades shelter in foxholes, but he abandons cover to stay above ground – screaming wildly and waving his fist at the enemy.

Ernst Simmel, a physician and self-trained psychoanalyst at a war hospital in Posen, took Oppenheim's claim one step further – with the help of Freudian theory. In his 1918 book, praised by Freud at the time he was writing *The Uncanny*, Simmel claimed that

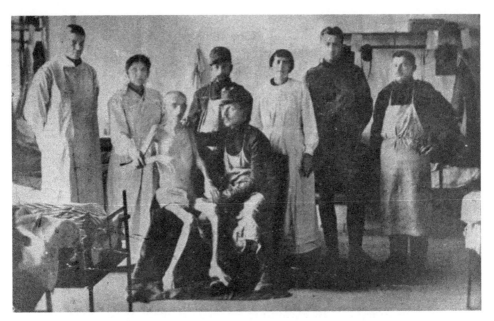

3. A soldier is rescued and brought to sick bay after being buried alive to the point of starvation. From Hirschfeld, *Sittengeschichte des Weltkrieges* (1930).

Verschüttung was the single most important cause of all war traumas. He even coined a medical term: "burial-alive neurosis" (*Verschüttungsneurose*).[21] Freud's praise for this man he did not yet know is logical when we consider Simmel's explicitly Freudian understanding of the word *Verschüttung*, which literally means "burial alive" but signifies also psychological "submerging." Freud had indeed written about *Verschüttung* repeatedly already in 1906, claiming that there is "no better analogy for repression, by which something in the mind is at once made inaccessible and preserved, than burial [*Verschüttung*] of the sort to which Pompeii fell a victim and from which it could emerge once more through the work of spades" (SE 9:40, GW 7:65).

Simmel takes Freud's analogy and applies it to soldiers who, like Jünger's comrade, have suffered this *Verschüttung* literally – not far from Simmel's field hospital. For Simmel, the double meaning of *Verschüttung* perfectly captured the genesis of war trauma. When the soldier was buried alive (*verschüttet*), often beneath dead friends and with sand blocking his nose and mouth, his ego too became submerged (*verschüttet*), resulting in the "sudden burial [*Verschütten*] ... of the personality-complex."[22] This prevented him from dispelling his fright through normal affective reactions, leaving it to descend intact into his "unconscious."[23] The fright settled there, as a repressed affect, which soon ossified into a neurosis. Enter here the psychoanalysts, who rushed to perform what Simmel called "mining work" (*Bergwerksarbeit*) – Freud's "work of spades," which complemented the military excavating of soldiers' bodies from trenches after explosions. Penetrating the patient's mind at its "highlands," Simmel's psychological miners located the gate to the mind's "depths" and descended to its "chasms" – where the man's ego had plummeted during his burial. Here, they discovered the affect that became "stuck" during the *Verschüttung*. Simmel describes the progression of this "mining [*Förderung*] of valuable material": he and his colleagues "mined deeply buried emotional complexes" until they "mined ... all causal materials to light."[24] By excavating this buried affect, these wartime analysts could save the man – just as Freud had done in peacetime.

The war thus gave new urgency to Freud's 1906 metaphor of *Verschüttung*, and this led to authors employing it in literature after the war. Not only does Freud evoke this image of burial alive in *The Uncanny*, so does Hugo von Hofmannsthal two years later in his play *Der Schwierige*. The drama is set shortly after the war, with the protagonist, a former soldier, plagued by his experience of being buried alive in his trench. When he curses his trauma as this "Verschüttetwerden," his female interlocutor knows exactly what he means, and she tries to help.[25] His body has been rescued, but as both he and she know, his trauma has remained submerged – leaving him unable to speak at key moments. The plot turns on precisely whether she can help him to excavate this trauma and – through this mining work – heal his psyche.

Kafka likewise recalls this trauma in "The Burrow" (1923) by inventing a creature-protagonist who lives buried in a network of tunnels that Kafka labels a "trench" (*Graben*). Partially inspired by Kafka's visit to a replica trench in 1915 and his work with injured war veterans, "The Burrow" restages soldiers' fears of being *verschüttet* by enemy mines – as I discuss in chapter 3. Kafka's creature develops a typical war strategy when he says he will collapse his series of trenches through an "Erdverschüttung," a term rarely used today but which, during World War I, denoted "burial by a fall of earth" (N2 625). The aim was to create an explosion that would entomb the enemy. When Freud cites "Erdverschüttungen" – and again, later, "burial under falls of earth" (*Verschüttung*) – as a primary cause of war trauma, he is referring to this tactic (SE 23:184, GW 17:111).[26] Kafka's protagonist plans to use it. He will cause an "Erdverschüttung" that will either kill his enemy or, as Simmel, Hofmannsthal, and Freud insisted, leave him brutally traumatized. If he were to do this, the creature would generate his own doppelgänger: another being who creeps beneath the earth in a permanent state of paranoia, another living metaphor for *Verschüttung*.

This trauma would have been repeated on a second level for postwar readers. Descriptions of burial alive had indeed seemed uncanny from Edgar Allan Poe onward. But, as Freud argues, they had now become the "most uncanny thing of all." For in his time burial alive combined ancient fears and desires (including the fantasy of returning to the womb) with a vision of entombment so contemporary and raw that it was almost unspeakable.

In the paragraph from *The Uncanny* immediately following Freud's reference to burial alive, he mentions the war again, this time remarking on his intellectual isolation during "the World War" (*des Weltkrieges*) (U 244, Ug 258). Despite this isolation, Freud was able still to get his hands on some foreign literature, specifically an issue of the English *Strand Magazine.* Here, he found the above-mentioned story that produced in him an "uncanny feeling" that was "quite remarkable" (U 244–5). Although Freud does not name this tale, he describes it sufficiently for us to be able to find it in a 1917 issue of the magazine. This issue's opening story already foregrounds the war – a "Hun" shouts "Gott strafe England" – and similar imagery looms over the entire volume, through to the story that affected Freud so deeply.

Entitled "Inexplicable," its plot is simple: A young couple moves into a house whose previous owner left behind a table inlaid with decorative alligators. Soon, the couple notices a stench, and the husband trips over an object slithering around his ankles (some loose carpet, he thinks). When the husband's friend, Jack Wilding, joins the couple for dinner, the normally mild-mannered Wilding begins to sweat, turn grey, twitch, and stutter. He claims that the house's odour reminds him of the alligator swamp in New Guinea in which he had just lost a comrade. The husband dismisses Wilding's "association of ideas," but Wilding remains haunted by this "waking nightmare" of New Guinea for the remainder of the evening.[27] When Wilding leaves the next day, the husband and wife seem, like the soldier's mother in *Nerves*, to become infected by his trauma: they too begin to see alligators. Panicked, they spend the night elsewhere, and, the following morning, the husband burns the carved table. The alligators miraculously do not return. The wife – also the story's narrator – says that this entire experience remains "inexplicable" to her. She closes with a challenge to the reader: "Does any explanation of it all occur to you?"[28]

Although Freud does not respond directly to the wife's challenge, we can see a military subtext that would have interested him. "Inexplicable's" pre-story – the death of Wilding's friend – occurs in New Guinea, part of which Germany still ruled at the onset of the war, and about which Freud would have read when the Australians defeated the Germans there in the 1914 battle of Bita Paka. New Guinea's military background becomes explicit in a drawing that accompanies Wilding's flashback. Outfitted in tropical helmet, boots, and rifle, Wilding walks across a bridge while his comrade is snatched to his death by the "loathsome brutes" (figure 4).[29] Unlike the man-eating brutes from Conrad's *Heart of Darkness* two decades earlier, Wilding's reptiles refuse to be "exterminated." Rather, they take revenge on the invaders. We see here the political unconscious of the story: England's sons will die in their colonial wars. If they return at all, it will be as traumatized veterans like Wilding. And these veterans' traumas will infect the home front. At the moment Wilding finishes telling his tale, he flails spastically to the ground, and this fit causes a "cloud of uncanny, shuddering sensations" to creep over the narrator.[30] She and her husband now see the alligators as well. Even though the alligators finally disappear when the husband burns the table, he knows that this incineration will not end the haunting: "Matter never dies," he says; and this smoke is "doing some useful turn elsewhere."[31]

This pestilent smoke that spreads "elsewhere," from person to person and place to place, made its way to Vienna and the Freud

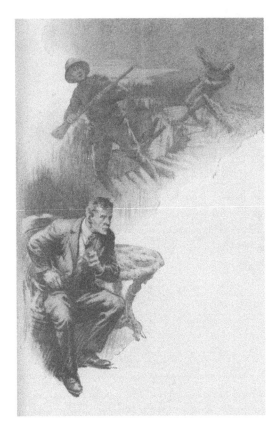

4. Wilding's flashback of his comrade being killed in the 1917 *Strand* story that gave Freud an "uncanny feeling."

family home, where it likely caused similar sensations. In 1917, two of Freud's own sons were fighting in Austria-Hungary's colonies: Martin Freud in Galicia and Ernst Freud in Slovenia (figure 5).[32] Freud hinted at worries about his sons already in his 1915 "Thoughts for the Times on War and Death"[33] and, in that same year, dreamt recurrently of them dying. He was especially shaken by his "prophetic dream" on the night of July 8, when he saw "very clearly … the death of my sons, Martin first."[34]

Three years later, in 1918, after being "without news of our son on the front for over a week," Freud had a distressing dream in which he unexpectedly finds his son returned home – strangely out of uniform and hidden away in a small storeroom. The son is climbing up on a basket:

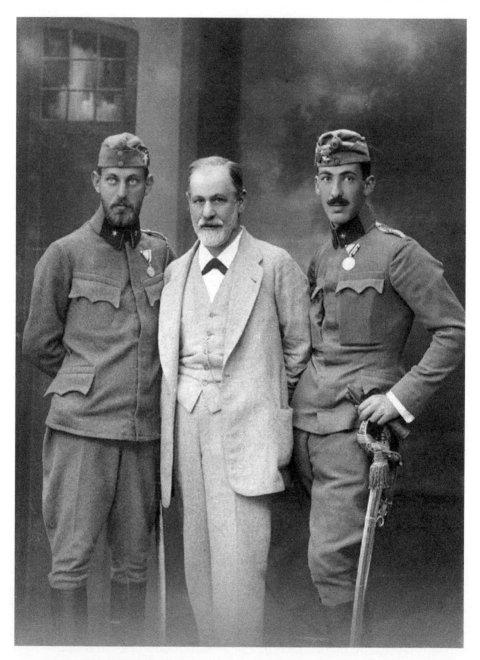

5. Freud in 1916 with his soldier sons, Ernst (left) and Martin, at home on
leave. Photo: Carl Ellinger. Library of Congress.

[My son] climbed up on to a basket that was standing beside a cupboard, as though he wanted to put something on the cupboard. I called out to him: no reply. It seemed to me that his face or forehead was bandaged. He was adjusting something in his mouth, pushing something into it. And his hair was flecked with grey. I thought: "Could he be as exhausted as all that?"

When Freud adds this dream to *The Interpretation of Dreams* in 1919, contemporaneously with *The Uncanny*, he interprets his son's "climbing" as its opposite: his "falling," or dying at war. Freud thus ignores a vitally troubling aspect of the dream – that the son is not dead but rather caught, uncannily, between life and death. What is more, Freud's soldier-son, like Wilding, bears symptoms whose provenance could not have been a mystery to Freud: head injury, premature greying, exhaustion, muteness, and fidgeting fingers. Freud even states that his dream-son's changed hair colour reminds him of his real-life son-in-law, whose hair had turned grey after being "hit hard by the war" (SE 4:559–60). But this does not lead Freud, or his readers, to state the obvious.[35] His soldier-son is not dead but traumatized, apparently by a war injury: confused, unable to speak, nervous, and lacking the motor skills to master the tasks of daily life.[36]

Just as this traumatized soldier appears but is not named in Freud's dream, so too does he remain silently at hand throughout *The Uncanny*. Immediately before Freud cites the uncanny fear of being buried alive, the "World War," and the popular story about the war ("Inexplicable"), he mentions the uncanny effect of "epilepsy," whose symptoms wartime psychiatrists likened to those of shell shock (U 243).[37] He then goes on to compile a list of the generally uncanny features that appear on human bodies:

Dismembered limbs, a severed head, a hand cut off at the wrist, as in a fairy tale of Hauff's, feet which dance by themselves ... – all these have something peculiarly uncanny about them, especially when, as in the last instance, they prove capable of independent activity in addition. (U 244)

No European reader would, in 1919, have associated these disjointed, severed, shaking bodies solely with fairy tales. When Freud moves in succession from E.T.A. Hoffmann's dolls, which are both "human being[s]" and "automaton[s]," to clairvoyant contact with "the departed," to the fear of the dead returning, to epileptic,

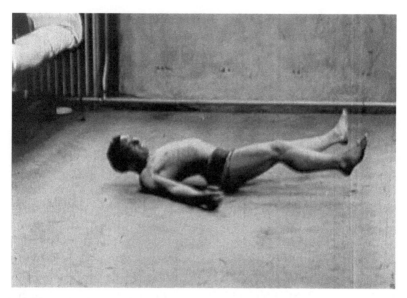

6. A "Kriegszitterer" (war shaker) in an English military hospital, 1917–18. Still from hospital footage. British Pathé.

dancing, amputated bodies, to the dread of burial alive, and to a British story about a traumatized soldier returning home, his readers would, like Wilding, have had an "association of ideas." But these would have led them well past fairy tales: to the dismembered "war cripples" (*Kriegskrüppel*) painted by the front veteran Otto Dix (see this book's cover) and to Oppenheim's war-shakers (*Kriegszitterer*), whose feet "danced by themselves" in Freud's Vienna and Wilding's London (home of Virginia Woolf's shell-shocked Septimus Smith) (see figure 6). The rhetoric of the *Kriegszitterer* thus assumes, within *The Uncanny*, its own contagious logic.

This latent presence runs through even the most well-known part of Freud's essay: his interpretation of Hoffmann's "The Sandman." The Sandman's mysterious night visits to the protagonist Nathanael's home culminate in what both Freud and Hoffmann call a traumatic "explosion" (*Explosion*), as discussed in chapter 1. A "fearful detonation, like the firing of a cannon," Hoffmann expounds, causes the death of Nathanael's father. For Freud, this produces in Nathanael the specific fear of losing his eyes and, by extension, his penis. This fear initially seems to have nothing to do with the war until we remember that both enucleation and castration were thoroughgoing fears of front soldiers. Shrapnel-induced enucleation was so frequent that the sudden dearth of German cryolite glass, used to make glass eyes, forced Allied medical officers to search for alternatives;[38] and there were so many castrations from explosions that a single German medical article cited 310 cases, along with anecdotes about the men being labelled "Karlchen ohne" ("Charlie without").[39] The sexologist Magnus Hirschfeld even created a specific medical category for these "War Eunuchs" in his *Sexual History of the World War*.[40]

Such war castrations appeared throughout postwar literature. Ernst Toller's 1923 expressionist play, *Hinkemann* (translated as *Brokenbrow*) and Hemingway's 1926 *The Sun Also Rises* present literally castrated protagonists. These characters symbolized the emasculated war veteran who returned from the front to find himself cuckolded and, in Germany, disrespected as a loser. Putting a castrated, humiliated veteran on stage sparked nationalistic outrage in Germany; Nazis and other völkisch groups protested the premieres of *Hinkemann* in Leipzig, Dresden, and Berlin.[41]

Although the war did not generate Freud's ideas on castration, it could have influenced his thoughts on Nathanael – especially if we consider that it was not actual injuries to genitalia but the *fear* of such injuries that, according to Freud, reactivated infantile anxieties. Like many of his colleagues in psychiatry,[42] Freud argued that "fright" played a significant role in the creation of all war neuroses and, what is more, that injured soldiers were actually less likely to develop these neuroses than were uninjured ones (SE 18:12). The most famous example of what psychiatrists called fear-based "hysterical blindness" was Lance Corporal Adolf Hitler, who supposedly received this diagnosis after the British pelted his division with mustard gas in October 1918.[43] Wilhelm Stekel, an early follower of Freud and a military psychiatrist treating shell-shock victims, claimed that "hundreds of thousands" of otherwise uninjured men were suffering from castration hysteria: neurotic "Kriegsimpotenz" (war-induced impotence). Like the narrator in "Inexplicable," Stekel uses the language of contamination to describe how this hysteria developed. *Kriegsimpotenz* was part of the "bitter fruit" sown by the war; this fruit was "poisoning" or "contaminating" (*vergiften*) more and more men. This contamination, Stekel warned, had taken on epidemic proportions. It was a public health risk that would eventually affect all of "humanity."[44]

We may not interpret the anxieties of an 1815 fictional civilian, Nathanael, as if he were a World War I soldier, but we can see how Hoffmann's descriptions in "The Sandman" of cannon fire, military cover, cries of woe, choking smoke, and distorted corpses recall Hoffmann's own "Great War": the Napoleonic battles in Prussia and Saxony, specifically the 1813 Battle of Dresden, which Hoffmann witnessed. As I argued in chapter 1, Hoffmann's copious writings about this battle predicted Nathanael's experiences often verbatim – revealing that major aspects of "The Sandman" are direct reworkings of Hoffmann's war experiences. More than this, Hoffmann describes in both his war notes and "The Sandman" a form of trauma that prefigured the "shell shock" of World War I: the "wind-of-the-cannonball" (*vent du boulet*) syndrome, which left soldiers with mysterious anxieties and phobias when shells passed nearby yet did not hit them. After nearly being hit, both Hoffmann and Nathanael suffer from the same psychological symptoms, feeling extremely "anxious" (Dv 806, Sg 19). Hoffmann calls this "one of the most remarkable days of my life." When later visiting the gruesome battlefield, strewn with maimed bodies, he gives us a clue as to how this experience will colour his nightmarish fictions: "What I have so often seen in dreams has come true – in a dreadful way – mutilated disjointed humans!!" (T 471).

Because Hoffmann's war experience reappears in his description of Nathanael, and because Freud wrote *The Uncanny* in the shadow of his own war, an otherwise anachronistic reading suggests itself. Might Freud and his contemporaries have seen in the traumatized Nathanael aspects of World War I soldiers – especially their own traumatized sons? This potential conflation of the Great War with the Napoleonic Wars reveals itself in a monumental typographical error and Freudian slip from Freud's 1920 legal memorandum on the treatment of the war neurotics. He and his colleagues met for a conference on shell shock, he writes, near the end World War I:

in "1818" (SE 17:215n1). Just as the Battle of Dresden was still powerfully present for Hoffmann two years after the fact (in 1815), the Napoleonic trauma remained with the fathers of the Great War a full century later. The postwar of 1918 senses the haunting return of the postwar of 1818. War trauma is contagious not just from body to body but also from past to present – and not only in the classical Freudian sense of childhood traumas infecting adulthood.

Nathanael's resemblance to the Great War neurotics treated by Stekel now comes into relief. Like these soldiers, Nathanael emerges from the cannon explosion symbolically castrated: he is incapable of having romantic relations with his fiancée. What is more, he acquires the hysterical idea that he has been amputated, like a soldier hallucinating after a shelling or a *Verschüttung*. The Sandman has "unscrewed my hands and feet," Nathanael cries. Typical also of trench soldiers, Nathanael blacks out after his traumatic experience. He has an abrupt convulsion, then feels nothing more, then awakens long afterwards, "as if from the sleep of death." Here and for the remainder of the story, Nathanael's symptoms resemble those of a traumatized soldier, whether from the Napoleonic Wars or World War I. Specifically, his bouts of twitching, shaking, and leaping prefigure the *Kriegszitterer* from 1914 to 1918. In the end, just before he commits suicide, Nathanael screams twice, "Feuerkreis!," which suggests a military "circle of gunfire." It recalls particularly the one that Hoffmann endured during the allied encircling of Dresden.

This is not to say that Nathanael's trauma is purely material, caused by the warlike explosions in his home. As Freud insists, Nathanael might have fantasized the evil Sandman/father out of infantile fears. But we do see here how an external event – the Battle of Dresden – can complicate early psychoanalysis's certainty about the etiology of trauma. First, the battle makes us question whether Nathanael's symptoms issue from castration anxieties at all. This, in turn, unsettles the general psychoanalytic conviction that infantile sexual complexes are the source of all trauma. This problem was not lost on Freud and his disciples, who faced precisely this dilemma when diagnosing the war neurotics. Stekel, Simmel, Sándor Ferenczi, and Karl Abraham were all military physicians who witnessed cases of shell shock and who, like Freud, asked: if the causes of all neuroses were psychological and sexual, then what about the undeniable power of the brutal "event" of battle?[45] (Infantile sexual trauma is of course also an "event," but even here Freud had minimized its importance, focusing instead on the child's fantasies already during his 1897–8 drawback from his seduction theory – well before writing *The Uncanny*.)

Freud's followers generally came down on the side of doctrine, with Ferenczi presaging Freud's hypothesis that shell shock was only a precipitating cause: it chaotically "unbound" sexual energies in people whose psychic systems were already not well "cathected" – often due to neurotic fantasies from childhood.[46] But Freud admitted that such theories were only speculations and that the war neuroses might indeed refer back only to this brute event of battle – specifically, because of submicroscopic brain damage that the battle might have caused. When the "strength of a trauma exceeds a certain limit," Freud confesses, "this factor [psychic hypercathexis] will no doubt cease to carry weight" (SE 18:32). Freud admits with chagrin that his position is now sounding like that "old, naïve theory of shock" that focused on the "effects of mechanical violence" (18:31). Yet Freud is also voicing here his own lifelong suspicion, beginning with his 1890s work on hysteria and reappearing now during the war, that a material substrate might indeed be lurking beneath all psychic illness.[47]

Freud's sense that there must be a physical source connects him to the medical tradition going back to Hoffmann and the Napoleonic Wars, when doctors assumed that hysterical soldiers had suffered inner ear damage from passing shells: the "wind-of-the-cannonball" syndrome. After this, they insisted that traumatized railway travellers had neurological injuries known as "railway spine," "railway brain," and, in Oppenheim's 1889 terms, a "molecular rearrangement" in the cerebrum.[48] Today's neuropsychologists similarly contend that traumatic symptoms must have a physical counterpart, although the majority of PTSD patients do not have brain lesions that can be detected through imaging. Scientists cite instead biochemical damage – "biological reactions" or "dysfunctions" of the brain – yet even here they waver on whether these are the causes or the effects of the symptoms.[49] The philosopher Catherine Malabou celebrates such neuropsychological research, claiming that we now know that "all traumas … are accompanied by brain damage."[50] But the psychiatrist and medical historian Esther Fischer-Homberger warns against trumpeting too quickly what we think we know about biology and trauma. Her sober genealogy of trauma from the nineteenth century onward puts such scientific certainties in perspective, reminding us that neurology has always maintained to have found *the* physical source. Today's "brain lesions" and "biological reactions" might indeed one day line up behind "railway spine," "railway brain," and "molecular rearrangement" in the awkward annals of the history of science.[51]

Freud intuits this and thus questions his own desire to locate a singular mechanical cause, sensing that there still must also be an infantile psychosexual source. In his 1919 introduction to the volume *Psycho-Analysis and the War Neuroses*, he sketched out how one might find this by connecting the war neuroses to conflicts in the ego, narcissism, and the "narcissistic libido." But he admits that such a theory is only provisional, awaiting the outcome "of our investigations." Although Freud is typically hopeful – "The theoretical difficulties standing in the way of a unifying hypothesis of this kind do not seem insuperable" – he must, for the time being, concede what he had said earlier in the introduction. Such a theory "has not yet been proved" (SE 17:209–10, 208).

Freud never does prove this connection between the war neuroses and sexuality, but he does make a fragmentary attempt in *Beyond the Pleasure Principle*, whose first draft he likewise completed in the spring of 1919. This attempt appears disjointedly in two distinct paragraphs separated by a couple of pages, but one can still glimpse here aspects of a theory similar to the one explored fictionally by J.G. Ballard in *Crash* (1972). In the second of these paragraphs, Freud argues that all motion – from rocking on a parent's knee to riding in a railway train – can produce "sexual excitation." The mechanical "violence" generated by a railway crash or a bomb explosion incites this same excitation, but this is now combined with "anxiety." Freud refers here back to the first of the two paragraphs: to the "preparedness" of the victim's psychic system for such an excitation. If his system is highly "cathected" – able to "bind" new, strange energies coherently into psychic patterns and narratives – then the mechanical violence will not result in a neurosis. Likewise, if this violence results in a physical injury, the victim will successfully bind these energies to his worries about the wound (18:33, 31). But if the victim has no injury and a poorly cathected psyche, the sexual-anxious energy will circulate chaotically, not bound to any object or idea. The result is neurosis. Freud's intervention peters out here. Although scholars have made ingenious attempts to reconstruct it more fully,[52] the fact remains that Freud never did, and he never believed that he had satisfactorily "proved" his speculations.

This lack of proof was no small matter. For war neurosis was the most pressing psychiatric problem of Freud's day and an urgent matter of national interest. As the number of shell-shock victims grew, both the Allied and Central Powers had to figure out ways to cure these victims and get them back to the front. This job went to psychiatrists in military hospitals, where the suspicion grew that many were faking. A "battle over simulation" (*Simulationsstreit*) that had hit its first high point in the 1880s and 1890s now raged again in psychiatric circles, especially at the 1916 "War Conference" of German neurologists.[53] Many psychiatrists were convinced that the majority of victims were malingerers, and they administered high-voltage electroshock treatments that rendered a cure worse than the disease. Soldiers fled back to the front. Some such psychiatrists faced charges after the war for "violations of military duty"; the 1920 legal memorandum that I cited above was part of Freud's own expert testimony at one of these inquiries (SE 17:211).

Freud claims that the Central Powers also considered employing psychoanalysis in the war effort. During the September 1918 Psycho-Analytical Congress in Budapest, high-ranking officials "promised" to establish treatment centres near the front (SE 17:207). Researchers have not yet found a document to corroborate Freud's claim (based on Ferenczi's account of a conversation with the chief medical officer of the Budapest Military Command),[54] but even if Freud exaggerated the state's interest, the point remains that he realized the importance of the war neuroses for psychoanalysis – as both opportunity and crisis. For just after citing this promise in his introduction to *Psycho-Analysis and the War Neuroses*, Freud reports that "the opponents of psycho-analysis" have already jumped on his failure to immediately connect the war neuroses to sexuality. This, his enemies triumphantly claimed, had "disproved" once and for all psycho-analysis's doctrinal basis (17:208).

Freud was thus fighting a war within a war in spring 1919 when he wrote the introduction to *Psycho-Analysis and the War Neuroses*, *Beyond the Pleasure Principle*, and simultaneously, as revealed in a May 12 letter to Ferenczi, *The Uncanny* (SE 17:218). In this strange, para-psychoanalytic text, Freud envisions, however unconsciously, the surreal aspects of shell shock that had exceeded his clinical work – specifically when, after discussing "The Sandman," he describes the characters in "Inexplicable." As in his memorandum on the war neurotics and Hoffmann's description of Nathanael, Freud begins with "motor disturbances": the characters in "Inexplicable" often "stumble" over things in the "dark" (17:212, U 245). Freud repeats here almost verbatim the language of the narrator, who says that the twitching Wilding "stumbled" over a "dark shape." Freud's "stumble" repeats Wilding's "stumble" and, more important, cites the story's specific connection between uncanniness and the war neurotic. Immediately after Wilding's fall, the narrator employs – for the only time – the word "uncanny," thereby linking Wilding's New Guinean flashback to uncanniness itself.[55]

The source of the uncanny in "Inexplicable" is the same as in this entire section of *The Uncanny*. The traumatized body returns from war and shocks civilians on the home front. Just as Freud is not fully aware of this connection, the narrator-wife of "Inexplicable" admits in strikingly Freudian terms that she too is unable to state the obvious, to recognize what she knows to be true. She can perceive Wilding's experiences only from a great psychic distance, from "the depths of my subconscious self."[56]

Why can Freud, too, perceive these experiences only in his subconscious self? As is often the case with his own repressions, Freud hints at the answer: he might have suppressed the war neurotic from *The Uncanny* because of guilt. He had, like so many fathers, uncritically sent his sons off to war.[57] More than this, he had wished for his son to die, as he admits in the interpretation of his wartime dream – because of "the envy which is felt for the young by those who have grown old." The fact that Freud's dream son is not dead but half-alive and traumatized only increases the guilt. The half-living trauma-tized son, unlike the dead one, never allows the father to complete what Freud calls the "painful" yet clean process of leave-taking (SE 4:560). This son remains forever in the Freud family's psychic store-room, threatening them – in their guilt – just as the dead loved one in Freud's 1915 essay threatened the survivors: Freud's son becomes that same vengeful "evil demon" that is "to be dreaded" (14:294).

In the context of the war neuroses, this revenge against the guilty takes the form of an infection – as we see in "Inexplicable." Immediately after the narrator calls Wilding's hysteria "uncanny," she learns that her otherwise sensible servants have become "in-fected" by Wilding's "panic-fear"; they too begin to see the alligators, sob madly, drop trays, and utter "hysterical" screams. Her husband assures his wife that the servants have only been contaminated by the "notions" of others. But this statement turns out to be truer than he had wished. For his wife, too, now sees dark shapes along the ground, and he, like Wilding, trips over one. He now even seems to become Wilding, the traumatized solider. He cries out, using "the very words Jack [Wilding] had used."[58]

In the section of *The Uncanny* following this discussion of "Inexplicable," Freud emphasizes this fear of contagion – through the "doppelgänger," who, as he had claimed earlier, causes us to "identif[y]" ourselves "with someone else" and, in so doing, lose our sense of self (U 234, Ug 247). In this same post-"Inexplicable" sec-tion, Freud relates a personal anecdote: he is in a train's sleeping compartment when the door to the adjoining bathroom flies open. An elderly man in a dressing gown approaches. Assuming that this man is confused and has lost his way, Freud jumps up to set him right, only to realize that the intruder is "nothing but my own reflection in the looking-glass on the open door." This shock reminds Freud that he still actually believes that he has a double and, what is more, that he believes this double to be "unheimlich" (U 248n1, Ug 262n1).

Freud's addled "doppelgänger" fits into the hidden series of trau-matized figures in *The Uncanny*. By appearing to Freud in a mirror, this man, like these figures and all doppelgängers, reveals that our ego has not "marked itself off" as sharply from others as we had thought

(U 236). This insight is especially ominous in the case of war neuroses and other traumatic neuroses, which seemed to disconnect themselves from actual injuries and move, like a virus, from one person to the next. Freud knew this first-hand, having spent much of his life stricken by "railway phobia" (*Eisenbahnphobie*) – a close relative of *Eisenbahnneurose* (railway neurosis), the standard German translation of "railway spine" (F 392, Fg 430).[59] Like most contemporaneous trauma theorists, Freud likened railway neuroses to war neuroses (SE 17:211),[60] and he understood that both could be contagious. When Freud says he lives in constant "fear of the next train accident," he knows that he fears both a physical injury *and* the fear itself: his fear could get worse by observing others' symptoms and fears. He can still live and work with his railway phobia, claiming once even to have "overcome" it, but a further infusion of anxiety – whether around trains or war – might turn *him* into the man in the mirror (F 262, 285).[61]

This danger becomes writ large in the anecdote's narrative perspective. Freud's apparently healthy ego ("I") attempts to heal the befuddled doppelgänger ("him"): "Jumping up with the intention of putting *him* right, *I* ..." But "he" refuses to let "I" put him right – remaining instead, like Wilding and Freud's dream-son, dogged in his confusion. Unable to straighten out this "he," the "I" gets drawn further into "his" bewilderment until realizing, "to my dismay," that "I" am the same as "he": "he" is "nothing but my own image." Yet even this knowledge – that "he" is part of "I" – does not neutralize the spectral power of "him." Well after this actual railway incident, at the time of writing *The Uncanny*, Freud "still" recalls "*his* appearance" – as if this baffled, traumatized "he" had been carrying on a life of its own, parallel to and within Freud's "I" (U 248n1).

This fear of becoming the traumatized other registers likewise in the grammar of the final two sentences of Freud's reading of "Inexplicable." While describing the anxieties of the story's characters, Freud dramatically shifts the meaning of the German pronoun "*man*" – sometimes translated as "one" but ultimately more multivalent and semantically unstable than this English counterpart:

> they [*man*] stumble over something in the dark; they [*man*] seem to see
> a vague form gliding over the stairs – in short, we [*man*] are given to

understand that the presence of the table causes ghostly crocodiles to haunt the place ... It was a naïve enough story, but the uncanny feeling it produced was quite remarkable [*ihre unheimliche Wirkung verspürte* man *als ganz hervorragend*]. (U 244–5, Ug 258)

"*Man*" moves here from twice meaning "they" (the frightened, stumbling characters from "Inexplicable") to "we" (the readers of "Inexplicable") to a subject-mishmash so confusing that James Strachey deletes it entirely from the translation: "the uncanny feeling it produced was quite remarkable." But, contra Strachey, Freud does provide a subject for this final sentence. Again it is "*man*," which seems here to denote "one" but refers also to 'I' – to Freud – who tells us: "ihre unheimliche Wirkung verspürte man als ganz hervorragend," literally "one [or 'I'] sensed its [the story's] uncanny effect as quite remarkable."

Through this semantic shift from "they" to "we" to "I," Freud slips from the safe position of the outside observer to that of the neurotic soldier, Wilding, who also represents Freud's dream-son, "hit hard by the war." Given this blurring of subjects, it is not surprising that Freud, as the "*man*" who is now both doctor/father and neurotic/son, feels himself, too, to be falling: "One [*man*] stumbles over something in the dark." Simultaneously first and third person, the falling Freud now resembles the war neurotic. And he can no longer deny what he sees: "One [*man*] sensed" the "uncanny effect."

This uncanny closeness of the healthy man – the doctor – to the neurotic was a long-standing fear in the history of the traumatic neuroses. Because early researchers could not locate an organic cause, these disorders were deemed purely psychic and thus capable of striking anyone at any time. What is more, these ailments seemed to be contagious, like the bacteria – and the very idea of infectious disease – that Robert Koch discovered in the 1880s. Wilding's hysteria and Stekel's "war impotence" were both apparently transmissible, especially because of the hysteric's tendency to imitate.

With the appearance of the first war neurotics at the onset of hostilities, such contagion became a matter of national interest. Already in the winter of 1914–15, German military doctors such as

Kurt Singer claimed that traumatized soldiers could "contaminate" the healthy ones.[62] They warned against a "psychic epidemic."[63] Singer himself became more convinced as the war progressed, insisting in 1918 that "a single hysteric" is more dangerous "through contagion" than an enemy who kills "a dozen healthy soldiers."[64] The director of the Clinic for Psychic and Nervous Illnesses at Berlin's Charité Hospital, Karl Bonhoeffer, used the term "war-hospital hysteria" (*Lazaretthysterie*) to describe the theatrical milieu of the sick bay, where new arrivals witnessed their ward mates acting upon "delusions" until these healthy ones began, "more or less consciously," to impersonate the sick.[65] The psychiatrist against whom Freud supplied testimony, Julius Wagner-Jauregg, insisted that he and his colleagues, who had been charged with treating the war neurotics, faced "a kind of epidemic." "Hysteria is an infectious disease," Wagner-Jauregg continued, "we call that an epidemic, and these peculiar motor neuroses [of the war neurotics] are a hysterical epidemic that arises in wartime."[66]

The German War Ministry was convinced. Beginning in 1917, they established discrete military psychiatric facilities that kept neurotics separate from other casualties.[67] But even such quarantining did not work. Cases of war neurosis increased among new recruits who had not yet seen combat and even among civilians hundreds of miles from the front. This all seemed to confirm the hypothesis of "psychic contagion."[68]

This sense that even a civilian's or a doctor's rational "I" could be transformed into the neurotic's "he" adds a final layer to the secret story of the war neurotic in *The Uncanny*. As Freud hints on the last page, the closeness of the healthy person to the neurotic double is not just one of many aspects of uncanniness. It is the uncanny's essence. Freud retells here Herodotus's story of the thief escaping his captor – the princess – by handing her, instead of his own arm, an arm severed from a corpse. The princess would certainly have gone unconscious in fright, Freud tells us, but *we* do not find the story uncanny at all because "we put ourselves in the thief's place, not in hers." Uncanniness, Freud insists, is a matter of perspective – just as it was in "The Sandman," when Nathanael looked through Coppola's *Perspektiv* and the narrator toggled between ironic distance and Nathanael's point of view. We can only experience uncanniness when we surrender what Freud calls our "ironical" position and adopt that of the person experiencing the shock (U 252).

Freud claims this only for "the world of fiction," but we now see how it pertains to uncanniness in general (U 252). Like the war neuroses themselves, uncanniness always concerns *someone else's* trauma; more specifically, it describes the moment in which "our" perspective disappears into "theirs." Recent psychoanalytic theorists make similar claims about trauma in general – without noticing this kernel in *The Uncanny*. Françoise Davoine and Jean-Max Gaudillière show how children with traumatized parents become "the subject of the other's [the parent's] suffering, especially when this other is unable to feel anything."[69] Cathy Caruth speaks of the ever-present danger "of trauma's 'contagion,' of the traumatization of the one who listens." Trauma, like history, is "never simply one's own," and history is nothing other than "the way we are implicated in each other's traumas."[70] In post-World War I Europe, when the hysterical fear of contracting war neuroses was great, this giving way of perspective seemed all too likely. The neurotic's point of view could infect anyone, as in the grammar of psychoanalysis that I discussed in chapter 1: the "I" (the *Ich*, the ego) was in constant danger of contagion from the "he" or "it" (the *Er* or *Es*, the id).

This unconscious fear is what kept the war neurotic from being acknowledged – in society at large and in Freud's essay, which can merely hint at his existence, here again, on this last page. You grab at the arm of the man next to you, only to find that this arm has been severed from its body. Through his hidden presence, the traumatized soldier generates within Freud's *The Uncanny* precisely the "uncanny effect" that Freud finds so "remarkable." This effect impels us to understand uncanniness itself differently: as not just a personal trauma but also as a symptom, and diagnosis, of the repression of this trauma during the Great War.

This collective unconscious within *The Uncanny* accentuates the crisis that the war neurotics created for psychoanalysis. Freud's inability to address the war neurotic directly in *The Uncanny* speaks more generally to his inability to solve the etiological problem of shell shock, which led him ultimately to abandon the topic. After a flurry of activity in 1919–20, he returned to the topic only at the end of his life, in 1939 – and this time exceedingly briefly: as something that, he admitted, continued to "elude" psychoanalytic investigation (SE 23:184). Despite this apparent impasse, we can now see how *The Uncanny* allowed Freud, however unconsciously, to explore the para-psychoanalytic aspects of that shock which otherwise exceeded his clinical and legal writings. Writ large here are the surrealist anxieties emerging from ego lability, bloodthirsty alter-egos, and invisible contagions. We see too the technological black magic that Jünger described, after being bombed from far away on his first day of battle in 1914, as "a ghostly manifestation in broad daylight."[71]

Such ghosts spawned others. Just as the conscripted soldier's "peaceful ego" feared its own murderous "parasitic doppelgänger" – stimulating an internal conflict that contributed to war neurosis – so too was every ego (*Ich*) threatened by contagion from the internal and external other, the third person (Freud, SE 17:209; GW 12:323). And so too was every war, like the Great War, haunted by the one that preceded it, as in the covert presence here of Hoffmann's trauma in Dresden. The traumatized other, past and present, continues to call out to us, and we assiduously make our ears deaf. Through this "voice that cries out *to another*," Freud implies a bond between trauma and testimony; he never fully theorizes this relation, as Caruth correctly states,[72] but he does offer connected fragments of such a theory right here, in *The Uncanny*.

Freud shows us how we, like the narrator of "Inexplicable," know that *his* affliction could infect anyone: the doctors who attempt to treat it; the civilians who try to describe it; and the readers who long to understand it. Like the readers of Freud's Herodotus story, we ultimately do not take the other's perspective; her trauma and its contagion must be kept at bay. We construct a protective shield – itself a product of modernity – just as Gregor Samsa does, as we will see in the next chapter. And we, like Samsa, watch with surprise as uncanniness hits us again. For the all-too-familiar shocks of war, industrialization, and terror keep returning to us, even today. Yet we still insist that they are strange – *unheimlich* – manifestations of ghosts.

Chapter Three

Inexplicable Tears: Trains, Wars, and Kafka's Aesthetic of Indeterminacy

Franz Kafka's interest in the effects of modern machinery on the human body extends back to his early years as a business traveller and tourist, when he described the dangers of transportation technology. He wrote, for example, of unsafe automobiles: a 1911 traffic accident that he witnessed on a Parisian boulevard; lines of cars bumping into each other in *The Missing Person (Amerika)* (1911–12); an ominous bus rumbling over Georg Bendemann as he commits suicide in "The Judgment"; and the daredevil Munich sightseeing trip in the 1911 novel-fragment *Richard and Samuel: A Short Journey through Central European Regions*. Even more than automobiles, trains were for Kafka treacherous, not least because they almost doubled their speeds in his lifetime – reaching velocities of 100 kilometres per hour by 1910. As Karl Rossmann notes in *Amerika*, trains brought great noise and ferocity to the countryside: while walking across open fields and gentle hills, he hears trains "thundering" across "vibrating" – *sich schwingenden* – viaducts (figure 7).[1] Later in life, Kafka says that humanity invented such travel technologies for good reason: to encourage physical presence against the absence-sponsoring telegram and telephone. But trains and cars were devised "at the moment of crashing," both figuratively (the war against the media was lost) and literally: in the rush to bring people together "natural[ly]," humans had created machines to transport themselves at unnatural speeds.[2] Modern travel technologies were, constitutionally, accidents waiting to happen. And the possibilities of injury were endless.

Kafka begins documenting these possibilities already in his never-finished 1907 novel *Wedding Preparations in the Country*, where he

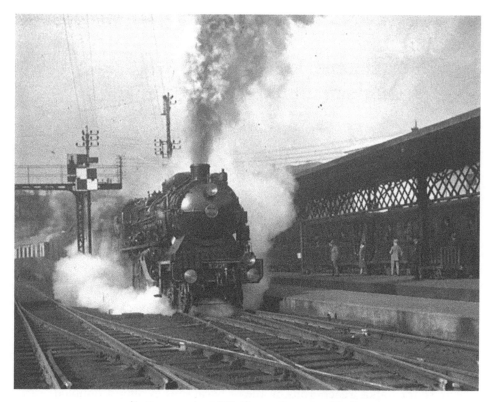

7. Steam train, 1927. Photo: Germaine Krull.

focuses primarily on the debilitating vibrations caused by trains. His hero, Eduard Raban, boards a train that pounds on the rails "like a hammer," and keeps "shaking" (*zitterte*) even after it stops (CS 64, 66; N1 35). Across from Raban sits a travelling salesman who bears the marks of this shaking. He can find no place to rest his vibrating arm, and his notebook "trembles" (*zittert*). This traveller then begins to shudder and cry for no clear reason: "not ashamed of the tears in his eyes," he presses his knuckles into his "quivering" (*zitterten*) lips (CS 64, 65; N1 31, 34). This trembling and sobbing man prefigures the post-WWI "war shakers" – *Kriegszitterer* – and echoes another traveller from *Wedding Preparations*: Raban's ghost-like double, the "clothed body," whom Raban usually sends on journeys in his stead and who now likewise "staggers," "stumbles," and "sobs" (CS 55).

Another early Kafkan traveller, Samuel from *Richard and Samuel*, has a similar experience in a train. The "vibration [*Zittern*] of the whole wooden, glass and iron structure," however pleasant at first, transmits itself when the train stops "through the whole of my sleep just as through the whole body of the train until it makes me wake up." This experience of being abruptly woken by a train, Samuel insists, constitutes a "shock." And like Raban's travelling salesman and the "clothed body" before him, Samuel eventually finds himself inexplicably at the point of tears (MP 293, 296; D 436).

Although these characters' symptoms have multiple causes – the travelling salesman has work worries, the clothed body must meet with the dreaded fiancée, Samuel is sexually frustrated – the fact that they appear repeatedly during or after train travel implies the influence of contemporaneous medical discourse. "Railway doctors" (*Eisenbahnärzte*) specializing in "railway illnesses" (*Eisenbahnkrankheiten*) and "railway health" (*Eisenbahnhygiene*) regularly saw similar bodies that quivered, shook, and trembled without apparent cause. Such illnesses resulted not only from crashes, doctors argued, but also from the fundamental inelasticity of trains. Beginning already in the 1860s, researchers reported that railway personnel and passengers were experiencing nerve and brain damage. The director of the Saxon Railways argued that the trains' constant "Erschütterungen" – meaning "shaking," "concussions," "shocks" – produced contractions and "trembling" (*Erzittern*) in the muscles and joints. These tremors ran up the legs and abdomen to the backbone and brain, creating swollen joints and obesity (from digestive disruption), as well as cerebral dysfunction and "brain congestion."[3] In a pamphlet on the railway's influence on public health commissioned by England's top medical journal, *The Lancet*, researchers claimed that the trains' continual "small and rapid concussions" produced a "commotion of the brain or spinal system of nerves." Even in milder forms, this commotion could result in a "disease" that – after "remaining a long time latent" – returned to afflict the nervous system.[4]

After the legal debate heated up in the 1890s about whether train-induced neuroses were physio- or psychogenic, researchers still insisted on the pathogenic importance of vibrations; the train's shaking seemed to transfer directly to the body. Doctors cited passengers who even continued to tremble in their sleep.[5] One German researcher argued in 1908, one year after Kafka began *Wedding Preparations*, that railway neurosis was – like seasickness – a "kineto-sis": brought on by "abnormal motion." In the case of the railway, this issued from "poor track construction" especially when the rails formed "severe curves." The resultant "shaking" (*zitter*[*n*]) often culminated in acute anxiety, including the "fear of death" and, in severe cases, "traumatic shock."[6]

In these early years of modern trauma theory, Freud similarly speculated in 1905 that the railway's mechanical "Erschütterungen" combined with fright to produce a "traumatic neurosis" (SE 7:202, GW 5:103). The British *Book of Health* had insisted on these neuro-ses' material substratum already twenty years earlier: "Man, for the time being, becomes a part of the machine in which he has placed himself, being jarred by the self-same movement, and receiving im-pressions upon nerves of skin and muscle."[7] Whereas horse-drawn carriages put wooden wheels on dirt, trains set steel upon steel, and this rigidity – in Kafka's words, "the collision of the rail points" (MP 293) – sent a series of small and quick concussions through the traveller's body. The "nervous-making shaking" nestled into the pas-senger's nervous system and left him quivering long afterwards.[8] As Kafka writes, the train's vibrations transmitted themselves "through the whole body of the train" into the body of the traveller.

To harden travellers against the shaking of the train, one German expert recommended sitting in a vibrating chair – a *Vibrationsstuhl* – before a journey.[9] But even this *Vibrationsstuhl* could not ultimately protect passengers, who still often ended up mirroring the vehi-cles that had transported them. In his popular book *Degeneration* (1892–3), the physician and social critic Max Nordau put a fine point on the conclusions of his medical colleagues. The railway was one of the greatest sources of modern nervous illness, especially hys-teria. And the main culprit was not the occasional dramatic crash of which one read in the papers but rather the "little shocks [*Erschütte-rungen*]" that were "not even consciously perceived." English doctors referred to nervous diseases as "railway spine" and "railway brain," Nordau argues, precisely because they issued from these industrial "Erschütterungen": from the shaking that travellers "constantly suffer in railway trains."[10]

Kafka's interest in this shaking appears not only in his early (pre-1912) stories, but also in his most famous tale, *The Metamorphosis* (1912), in which the protagonist, Gregor Samsa, travels the rails professionally. When Samsa transforms into a "monstrous vermin," he in fact assumes that he is suffering from "the torture of traveling" and has contracted an "occupational ailment of the traveling salesman" (M 4, 7). We should of course not simply accept Samsa's interpretation, for he misinterprets many things about himself. But we should ask why Kafka inserts this self-diagnosis at all. As I argue in this chapter, Kafka does this for two reasons. First, he aims to expose the deleterious effects of modernity – a task for which he is better suited than other modernists who delivered similar critiques. Of the great writers of his era (Joyce, Proust, Mann, Woolf, Eliot, etc.), Kafka was the only one to endure regular third-class rail travel for his work and the only one to see the inside of a factory; he visited shop floors regularly as a bureaucrat involved in workers' accident insurance claims and in connection with his family's own asbestos factory.[11] The second reason is complex, for Kafka is much more than a Zolaesque realist intent on criticizing industrial technology. He wanted to investigate how the legal and medical ways of speaking about trauma that he encountered at work related to his writing – specifically, to the problems of mimesis and truth at the essence of art.

Critics have long asserted that Kafka responds to this aesthetic problem with a poetics of indeterminacy, a "radical aesthetic intention" that Stanley Corngold defines as Kafka's clear-sighted awareness of writing's limitations and of the "opaque and impoverished" nature of the linguistic sign.[12] As convincing as this argument is, also with respect to subsequent scholarship,[13] it neglects the historical background of this radical intention. For Kafka's awareness of the impoverishment of the sign is not without context. His poetics of indeterminacy, I maintain, is at once literary and historical-political. It is a response to the *linguistic* aspects of Kafka's entire business of accident insurance: the medical-legal discourses surrounding train travel, the Balkan Wars, World War I, and the treatment of veterans after 1918. More specifically, I argue that Kafka is reacting to the medical-legal insistence that we locate a single material cause for the traumatic symptoms of modernity. Kafka's challenge begins in *The Metamorphosis* and intensifies in his later stories, where he eventually presents us with symptoms that seem to be completely disconnected from the physical world. In these stories, Kafka increasingly unmoors all of his language and metaphors from identifiable reference points – thereby producing a more specific form of indeterminacy, a poetics of trauma.

Kafka's awareness of the discourse surrounding train trauma is clear in the technological diction of his early heroes – the "action of the carriage springs," the "friction of the wheels," and the "vibration of the entire wooden, glass and iron structure" – and in *The Metamorphosis*, which builds on the train story in *Wedding Preparations* (MP 293). When Raban sent his "clothed body" travelling in 1907, he wanted to remain in bed and metamorphose into a "beetle" (CS 55–6). The widespread assumption that Raban prefigures Gregor Samsa neglects, however, an important distinction.[14] Whereas Samsa is explicitly a traveller, a "traveling salesman" or "commercial traveler" (*Reisender*), Raban unequivocally is not: "I have never traveled" (M 3, D 115, CS 45). From this perspective, Samsa has more in common with the sobbing travelling salesman (also a "Reisender") than he does with Raban (N1 31).

Kafka believed that his stories could "mediate" between one another: "The Judgment" and "In the Penal Colony" would be "two alien heads knocking violently at each other" if they did not have *The Metamorphosis* in the middle of them (L 126).[15] In this spirit, we can envision a similar internal conversation between *The Metamorphosis* and *Wedding Preparations*. *Wedding Preparation*'s earlier travelling salesman has now *become* Samsa, I maintain, playfully reconfigured by Kafka five years later. We learn already in the opening paragraphs of *The Metamorphosis* that Samsa has worked as a travelling salesman for exactly five years, coinciding with the time Kafka wrote most of *Wedding Preparations* (1907) to the year he wrote *The Metamorphosis* (1912). That Kafka was more than passingly interested in this travelling salesman from *Wedding Preparations* is evident in the man's unusually intimate relation to Raban. This travelling salesman looks the entire time intently at Raban, never once turning his face away, until Raban feels compelled to engage him in small talk. Then this traveller, like the clothed body before him, begins to shake and cry. If Samsa has a prequel cameo in *Wedding Preparations*, it is not as Raban's happily lounging, stay-at-home beetle but as this proto-hysterical travelling salesman, tossed about in a train that "beats on the rails like a hammer" (CS 64).

This supposition gains force when we learn that Raban – long seen as a cipher for "Kafka"[16] – cannot understand the business talk of this commercial traveller, claiming that "much preparation [*Vor-bereitung*] would first be required" (CS 64, N1 31). The "prepara-tions" for *The Metamorphosis* begin precisely here, on this 1907 train, with Kafka/Raban declaring his need to gain more knowledge of professional travel, which Kafka notoriously does during his five subsequent years of "maddening" business journeys to factory re-gions outside of Prague (LF 64).[17] While writing *The Metamorphosis*, Kafka uses the same noun that Samsa does – "Aufregung" (agita-tion, irritation, upset) – to describe his workaday woes, and Kafka's recurring complaints about professional travel mirror Samsa's (BF 102, D 116). Kafka too must repeatedly catch early trains: "Tomor-row I have to get up at 4:30 AM again" (LF 229). And Kafka too suffers from what Samsa calls "the torture of traveling": never sleep-ing enough, "eating miserable food at all hours," and always feeling alone (M 4). Consider, for example, Kafka's departure for a business trip to Leitmeritz just two days after completing *The Metamorphosis*: "off I march while it's still almost night, wander through the streets in the piercing cold – past the breakfast room at the 'Blaue Stern,' its lights already on but curtains still drawn" (LF 97).

A couple of months later, before a trip to Aussig, Kafka cannot sleep despite great weariness because he is haunted by visions of the very trains that will transport him: "trains came, one after another they ran over my body, outstretched on the tracks, deepening and widening the two cuts in my neck and legs." The trains of course do not actually slice him up. But they do exhaust him, to the point that he, like the "clothed body," sits soullessly at his hotel table "like a puppet" (LF 230). Beside himself for days with "sleepiness, exhaus-tion, and anxiety [*Unruhe*]," Kafka eventually even transforms into an animal, like Samsa: "What I bore on my body was no longer a human head" (LF 229–30, BF 346).

Business travel repeatedly gives Kafka this same anxiety (*Unruhe*). Consider again his trip to Leitmeritz, when he feels "all the time uneasy, all the time uneasy [*unruhig*]," and his journey to Kratzau, in the midst of writing *The Metamorphosis*: "There wasn't a single moment on the trip when I didn't feel at least a tiny bit unhappy" – especially during the train ride itself, when he felt "restless" (*unruhig*) from the moment it began (LF 97, 67; BF 171, 130). Worrying "that the trip may have harmed my story," Kafka concludes bluntly in a letter to Felice Bauer: "One shouldn't ever go away." Yet he soon finds himself threatened again by impending travel: "Oh God, another journey is in store for me" (LF 67, 89). It is, however, precisely these journeys that "prepare" Kafka – as Samsa later insists, "on his own person/body" (*am eigenen Leibe*) – for writing *The Metamorphosis* (M 18, D 136–7). Kafka awakens one morning five years after writing *Wedding Preparations* in "misery," dreading another beastly professional trip, only to invent a new story (LF 47). The "incubation" or "latency" period typical for train-illnesses and traumatic neuroses had begun five years earlier, in 1907, and ends now, with a young travelling salesman waking from "unsettling" (*unruhigen*) dreams to find himself pathologically transformed (M 3, D 115).[18]

The Metamorphosis begins precisely with this assumption that Gregor Samsa is "ill" from the same beastly rigours of professional travel that afflicted his author. His mother says, "Gregor is sick"; his sister asks, "Is something the matter with you?" (M 14, 6); and Gregor himself concludes that he has contracted an "occupational ailment of the traveling salesman." Gregor's symptoms tally with the findings of train-illness research from the earliest years onward, which claimed that five years of regular train travel would be dangerous to anyone – especially to commercial travellers, who were more susceptible to everything from "overexcitement" to premature aging.[19] Gregor's symptoms echo the railway doctors' descriptions, which included the same melancholia, anxiety, and involuntary muscle movements present in the travellers in *Wedding Preparations*. Gregor, anxious and dejected, can suddenly "not control" his limbs, which wave wildly "in the most intensely painful agitation [*Aufregung*]" (M 7, D 121). Researchers furthermore cited chronic fatigue as a symptom of railway illness,[20] and Gregor, like his author, complains repeatedly of "drowsiness," "exhaust[ion]," "weari[ness]," and "general fatigue" (*allgemeiner Müdigkeit*) (M 6, 18, 45, 30; D 153).

Doctors also discovered that victims of railway crashes and those simply afraid of crashes had "distressing and horrible" dreams. They woke up "suddenly with a vague sense of alarm," and were "unusually talkative" and "excited."[21] Such premonitions of modern trauma theory apply to Gregor, who suffers from "unruhigen" dreams. After waking, he remains silent at first, then explodes in nervously "insistent distressed chirping" that he "hastily blurts" out (M 6, 13).

Another regularly reported symptom of train travellers was failing vision caused by eye fatigue and blurring landscapes. Observers claimed that the human eye, accustomed to the leisurely pace of horse carriages – eight kilometres per hour – could not focus at the subsequent fifty (1840), sixty-five (1860), and one hundred kilometres per hour (1910) of trains.[22] The "incessant shifting of the adaptive apparatus by which [objects] are focused upon the retina" was particularly harmful to travelling salesmen, who "in the course of one day have to cast their eyes upon the panoramas of several hundreds of places."[23] Nordau made similar claims in 1892: "Every image that we perceive from the compartment window of an express train sets our sensory nerves and brain centers in action."[24] When Raban looks out of his "racing" train window in 1907, he sees only "lights flitting past," villages "coming toward us and flashing past," and bridges that appear to be moving: "torn apart and pressed together," or so "it seemed" (CS 64–5). These high-speed apparitions tire Raban's eyes and those of his fellow travellers. When Raban deboards, the others see him blurrily from the train window, as if the train were still "in motion" (67).

In 1912, the professional traveller Gregor Samsa similarly discovers his vision abruptly weakened: "From day to day he saw things even a short distance away less and less distinctly." Even the hospital across the street, which might have been the ill traveller's only hope, is now "completely beyond his range of vision." If Gregor hadn't known that he lived on a city street, he would have thought he was still looking out a train window. For he sees only a blur, where "the gray sky and the gray earth were indistinguishably fused" (M 32).

Like Gregor's failing eyesight, his "worrying about train connections [*Zuganschlüsse*]" jibes with medical claims: that the railway's ruthless punctuality caused debilitating psychological stress, especially because of travellers' lingering confusion about standardized time (M 4, D 116). Before the advent of the railways, every town had a slightly different time: Reading, for example, was four minutes later than London, but ten minutes ahead of Bridgewater. Because these differences did not allow for interregional timetables and often caused crashes, railway companies eventually introduced "railway time," which at first meant only that each company kept its own time, enforced by the originating conductor passing his watch to a new conductor at the next station. This too led to accidents, such that governments eventually instituted a uniform railway time. Not surprisingly, mix-ups between this new "railway" time and "local" time persisted – even after the introduction of international standard time (in 1893 in Germany and Austria-Hungary). Arthur Schnitzler's 1900 protagonist of "Lieutenant Gustl," for example, absurdly can't decide whether he should commit suicide at 7 a.m. "Vienna time" or "railway time" (*Bahnzeit*).[25]

Researchers from the mid-nineteenth through to the early-twentieth century claimed that many railway illnesses issued not primarily from industrial mechanics but from time's mechanization. The "fearfully punctual train" produced "excitement, anxiety, and nervous shock" in travellers.[26] In 1901, a German doctor reported that people who rushed to the station sweating and distressed were susceptible to "tooth or even facial pain, throat and lung catarrh."[27] Another warned in 1908 that the "hurry and agitation before departure" led people to eat in haste and so suffer "revolution-motions" in their stomachs on the train.[28]

This anxiety about missing trains runs through Kafka's fiction from *Wedding Preparations* all the way to the 1922 parable, "A Comment": "I was going to the railroad station. When I compared the tower clock with my watch, I saw that it was already much later than I had thought, I had to rush, the shock of this discovery made me unsure of the way" (K 161). Raban already experienced this same time uncertainty and "shock" during his 1907 walk to the station. His own watch is broken. A stranger tells him it is "past four," then he hears a clock strike quarter to five. A friend says that Raban has "plenty of time," but he is nonetheless certain that he will "miss the train." The friend now says that it is quarter to six, but the station clock only strikes this later, when Raban arrives. When the porter finally rushes him onto the train, Raban experiences the same excitement and heart "palpitations" that railway doctors attributed still in 1907 to punctuality fears – as already detailed by Dr. Alfred Haviland in his 1868 medical monograph about the railway, *Hurried to Death* (CS 54, 59, 60, 62).

Gregor suffers likewise from anxieties about missing trains, to the point that he spends his evenings obsessively perusing railway timetables. He recalls here his author, who speaks to Felice Bauer of "train-hours" and repeatedly of his debilitating personal "timetable": "[I can write] until 5 in the morning; no later, because my train leaves at 5:45"; "I have to leave at 6 tomorrow evening; I get to Reichenberg at 10, and go on to Kratzau at 7 the next morning"; and "before my trip to Aussig, I did not get to bed until 11:30 ... ; I still heard 1 o'clock strike, and yet had to be up again [to catch a train] by 4:30" (LF 95, 62, 230). On the morning of his transformation, Gregor similarly thinks comically only about the railway's pitiless punctuality, not about his physical state: "I'd better get up, since my train leaves at five" (M 5).

Railway time oppresses Gregor partially because it moves irrationally fast, as it did for Raban. After realizing that he has overslept and that it is already half past six, Gregor watches as the clock hands move uncannily quickly, continuing "past the half-hour" and, before his eyes, to quarter to seven (M 5). Like the clock in Fritz Lang's *Metropolis*, these accelerated hands parody global modern mechanized time. Gregor's clock continues to torment him for the following forty-five minutes, the entire duration of the first third of the story. To cite just a few examples: "the alarm clock had just struck a quarter to seven"; "'Seven o'clock already,' [Gregor] said to himself as the alarm clock struck again"; and "Before it strikes a quarter past seven, I must be completely out of bed" (6, 8, 9).

Gregor attributes this unforgiving timekeeping to the punctuality of trains: "The next train left at seven o'clock; to make it, he would have to hurry like a madman," and "even if he did make the train, he could not avoid getting it from the boss, because the messenger boy had been waiting at the five o'clock train" (M 5). Gregor's family, too, is obsessed with railway time: "Gregor, it's a quarter to seven," his mother asks, "Didn't you want to catch the train?"; his father yells, "Gregor, the manager has come and wants to be informed why you didn't catch the early train"; and his mother adds, "Believe me, sir, there's something the matter with him. Otherwise how would Gregor have missed a train?" (6, 11). Time slips by with each missed departure, and, as if Gregor didn't already know it, the chief clerk reminds him that time is money: "You make me waste my time here for nothing" (13). Out of joint with time, Kafka's always-prompt traveller loses his bearings: tormented by conscience for wasting only "a few hours" of the firm's time, Gregor is "driven half-mad" and becomes "actually unable to get out of bed" (10). When Gregor finally dies at the end of the story, he does even this according to the timepiece: "He remained in this state of empty and peaceful reflection until the tower clock struck three in the morning" (59).

Driven mad by railway time, Gregor is, as critics have noted, an alienated worker: a subject transformed into a Marxian object.[29] But it is vital to add that Gregor's objectification is amplified because of his job as a professional traveller. As Marx insists, transportation is the only industry where production and consumption occur "simultaneously"; that is, where the product – change of place – is consumed at the same time that it is produced, resulting in a commingling of labour and consumption.[30] Even though the traveller – unlike the conductors, stokers, and attendants – is not explicitly working, the machinery works on him. The train's vibrations and noise give the modern bourgeois his only direct experience of industry. In Gregor's words (coincidentally repeated by Wolfgang Schivelbusch in his book on the railway), the traveller experiences industrialization "am eigenen Leibe": on his own body.[31] It is as if consumers were to consume manufactured goods *inside* the factory. This comparison is especially apt for the non-upholstered third-class wooden benches on which Kafka sat (and Gregor as well, who undoubtedly travelled in the same class as his fellow *Reisender* from *Wedding Preparations*).[32] With production and consumption so unusually intertwined, the transport industry unmasked any remaining delusions about the autonomy of the bourgeois subject. As Marx writes, "humans and commodities" travelled together within the same "means of transport"; more explicitly than in other industries, humans became here "living appendages" to the machinery.[33]

Early train travellers from all political stripes agreed. Unlike the passenger in a horse carriage, who could see the natural sources of the horsepower and of the bumps and jerks, the industrial passenger knew neither how his vehicle functioned nor why it shook and clattered. The traveller was alienated and unaware, ultimately nothing more than a "package," a "bale of commodities," or, in the words of Joseph Maria von Radowitz, a "piece of freight."[34] Gregor Samsa becomes precisely such a commodity, a body transported from place to place for the profit of both his firm and his family. Gregor's father indeed has secretly been keeping part of Gregor's wages instead of using this to pay off his debts, thereby increasing the time that Gregor must spend travelling.

Gregor has perhaps tallied his own symptoms with us: fatigue, twitching muscles, uneasy dreams, nervous volubility, blurred vision, and psychological stress from timetables and alienation. For he now minces no words about his diagnosis. "The torture of traveling," "worrying about train connections," and being "day in and day out – on the road" have caused this traumatic "upset," these "agitations" (*Aufregungen*) (M 4, D 116). Gregor has "no doubt in the least" that he is suffering from this common "occupational ailment of the traveling salesman" (M 7). Scholars have ignored Gregor's claim, instead generally viewing his transformation as an externalization of an internal conflict: his desire to punish himself (for having usurped his father's role), his masochistic "self-hatred," or his latent "death drive."[35] This 'externalization' reading extends even to contemporary poststructuralist and post-Freudian readings, which see Gregor's transformation, for example, as a "becoming-visible" of the lack of a "consistent and dependable Other."[36] Even the rare critics who accept Gregor's insistence that he is "ill" do not follow his specific claim that this is an "occupational" ailment, one brought on by years of riding the rails.[37] Might it be time to take Gregor at his word?

But as with so many other possible interpretations of *The Meta-morphosis*, Gregor's own – and the one I have been presenting so far – is challenged by Kafka himself. This begins already in *The Metamorphosis*'s pre-story, *Wedding Preparations*, when Raban denies that his clothed body is diagnosable in any way. According to Raban, his body's first symptom ("staggering") "indicate[s] not fear but its nothingness." Raban does not simply refute the reading, "My 'clothed body' is pathologically scarred by train travel"; he refutes *any* such direct relation of a signifier ("staggering") to a signified ("fear"). The body points only to "nothingness." Its "stumbling," Raban continues, is furthermore not "a sign of agitation [*Aufregung*]." Like Gregor's hermeneutically resistant shell, Raban's "clothed body" is vehemently *not* a "sign." It does not "indicate" or "show": it "zeigt ... nicht" (CS 55, N1 18).

Indeed, as critics have pointed out, Kafka's bodies resist meta-phorical – and diagnostic – readings because Kafka's human tenors and material vehicles are labile. The metaphor is always in motion.[38] Gregor's transformation is unfinished: Is he an animal or is he our son? This question renders all interpretations of his body unstable. Because Gregor's body, like Raban's clothed body, cannot point to-wards a stable meaning – cannot function reliably as a "sign" – the reader is at an interpretative impasse. Why do Kafka's travellers stag-ger and stumble? Why do they cry? Why, in the most extreme case, do they metamorphose? Kafka's bodies deny our answers before we can formulate them.

But this problem of the opaque sign lies at the heart of fin-de-siècle trauma discourse, especially its legal branch. For Gregor, the confusion about his bodily symptoms leads him to fear the "health-insurance doctor" (*Krankenkassenarzt*), whose job resem-bles that of the deconstructivist critic: he must prove that the body is *not* a functioning sign, that it points to *nothing*. According to the feared *Kassenarzt*, nothing at all is causing Gregor's symptoms; he simply doesn't want to go to work, is "afraid to work" (work-shy, "arbeitsscheu") (M 5–6, D 119).[39] Gregor's dread of the *Kassenarzt* lends a legal-medical context to the long-standing literary prob-lem of Gregor's apparently unreadable body. As Kafka certainly knew, railway vibrations and crashes had already created many people who presented no physical injuries but nonetheless suffered breakdowns and were, like Gregor, "unable to work" (M 17). Because the German railways became legally liable for injuries after 1871 – almost single-handedly creating Kafka's profession of accident insurance in 1884 (1887 in Austria-Hungary) – the legal-medical debate about traumatic neuroses exploded by the fin de siècle.[40] Doctors now had to distinguish between the truly injured and what Gregor's *Kassenarzt* calls the "completely healthy" simulators (M 5).

The debate began already after railways became liable in England in 1864, and medical-legal doctrine initially followed John Erichsen's 1866 claim that victims of crashes or of shaking in trains were anatomically damaged. They had suffered lesions on their spinal column: the "railway spine" to which Nordau later referred.[41] Beginning in the early 1880s, after autopsies of spines proved negative, researchers argued that there was no spinal damage. They shifted the focus to the brain ("railway brain") and to what Hermann Oppenheim in 1889 influentially termed a "traumatic neurosis" of the cerebral cortex (see chapter 2). This move from spine to brain coincided with the replacement of Erichsen's theory of pathological anatomy with biochemical explanations. "Molecular rearrangement" or "functional disturbances" in the cerebral cortex affected "the psyche as well as the centers for motility, sensitiveness, and sensate functions."[42] Oppenheim's book led to immediate changes in German insurance law. The Imperial Insurance Office now deemed "traumatic neuroses" eligible for compensation.[43]

But because the molecular brain damage that Oppenheim cited was submicroscopic, doctors were not able to distinguish between the work-shy simulators and the truly ill. This led to an explosion of the already simmering battle around simulation – the *Simulationsstreit* – which reached its first apex in the 1890 Medical Congress in Berlin. Opponents of Oppenheim argued that all neurotic symptoms, even the telltale full-body shake, could easily be simulated. They claimed that over 25 per cent of all traumatic neuroses were faked.[44] Oppenheim countered by claiming that most of his opponents were insurance doctors (*Kassenärzte*) who, just as Samsa had feared, were in the pockets of big business – mostly the "railway."

They were "simulation hunters" (*Simulantenjäger*), who "saw simulation everywhere they looked."[45]

Enough doubt was shed on Oppenheim's "molecular" argument that the 1880s psychogenic theories of Herbert Page, Jean-Martin Charcot, Pierre Janet, and Paul Julius Möbius gained new momentum. Möbius argued that he would rather have testable psychological theories than Oppenheim's "labile molecules," for which no "demonstrable data" existed.[46] Although these researchers still held, more or less, to the likelihood of accompanying somatic trauma, they argued that Oppenheim's "traumatic neuroses" – which Charcot termed "traumatic hysterias" already in 1876 – could also be caused by ideas, suggestions, or fantasies.[47] Even before Freud de-emphasized his seduction theory in 1897, he likewise stressed the etiological importance of fantasy and psychic predisposition. Each patient's constitution and sexual and family history helped to determine whether a particular shock produced in them the profound disruption that caused hysteria.[48] Despite Freud's hopes of improving his patients' lives, this psychogenic theory did not help them financially. For the legal principle remained until the 1960s that only primarily physical injuries could be compensated.[49] Oppenheim's insistence on molecular damage thus remained vital for indemnification.

During this period, after the theorization of psychogenic trauma but before its legal acceptance, Kafka, a legal clerk at the Workers' Accident Insurance Institute, created a damaged body that had to submit itself to a *Kassenarzt* for interpretation. This *Kassenarzt*, even if he were benevolently inclined, could never find the somatic source necessary for legal compensation. Gregor Samsa has the typically hysterical body of his day: symptomatic but with an "undetectable pathological-anatomical substrate." This "submicroscopic" cause of his suffering is at once also the missing link; molecular damage could not be proven. In this way, the "ultramodern" medical language of hermeneutic undetectability[50] mirrors the postmodern literary-critical assertion of Gregor's "unreadability." But this interpretative language now develops significance beyond literary criticism's games of semiotic self-reference. Opaqueness points instead towards the traumatized body itself. Like the slanderous rumours swirling around travelling salesmen, Gregor's symptoms are only felt subjectively, on his own body – "am eigenen Leibe" – and can therefore never be "traced back to their causes" (M 18, D 136–7). His injured body is left only to make mute or garbled entreaties that are not even understood.

By the end of Gregor's story, the three boarders threaten to use his body as legal proof in a suit against his family, but the tragedy is that this same body cannot be used to supply evidence for itself. It cannot help doctors to uncover an original "cause" and therefore, perhaps, a cure. Even Gregor admits, despite his telltale symptoms of "railway illness," that his self-diagnosis will not convince the authorities. The *Kassenarzt* might not "be so very wrong" in assuming that he is simulating (M 6). And this is not just because it runs in the family (Gregor's parents and his sister invent "letters of excuse" at the end to get off of work) (62). Gregor's uncertainty lurks deeper. His claim that he is not sure whether he is simulating prefigures Freud's statement from 1920, "All neurotics are malingerers; they simulate without knowing it, and this is their sickness."[51] To rephrase this in the broader terms of my reading: we cannot know whether Gregor is suffering from a train-induced trauma, but we do know that he suffers from that same illness of suspected simulation that haunted all travelling bodies at the fin de siècle.

Even if railway trauma inheres precisely in diagnostic doubt, one could still object to my reading on the basis of Gregor's radical transformation, which parodies any imaginable case of traumatic neurosis. Gregor does not simply quiver, chatter nervously, and sleep badly; he becomes a giant insect. But if we look at Kafka's story in the context of his general interest in mechanized bodies from 1907 to 1914, we see a steady progression towards hyperbole that could explain such an overstatement. On the heels of the lightly damaged travellers from *Wedding Preparations* and *Richard and Samuel*, Kafka creates a commercial traveller who explodes medical orthodoxy. Travel "agitations" lead not only to uneasy dreams, fatigue, twitching muscles, and blurred vision, but to a complete metamorphosis.

The way is now clear for Kafka's exaggerated victim-bodies, as foreshadowed in the above-mentioned 1913 dream, where trains ran over his body. The 1914 "In the Penal Colony" creates such a body by reconfiguring the steam locomotives from *Wedding Prepa-rations* and *Richard and Samuel*. This new machine has "screeching" wheels that generate a thoroughgoing "Zittern": the apparatus "quivers [*zittert*] with very rapid, tiny vibrations, both from side to side and up and down" (K 38, 39; D 209). As in contemporary med-ical discourse about trains, this vibrating machinery reproduces it-self on the body: "Quivering [*zitternd*], it sticks its needles into the body, which is itself quivering [*zittert*] from the vibrations of the bed" (K 42, D 215). In Kafka's hyperbole, this body becomes wholly "transfigur[ed]" or even, in the case of the officer's "quivering" (*zit-ternd*) body, "murder[ed]" (K 48, 57; D 244).

Kafka's 1914 penal apparatus is not simply a train in disguise, but neither is it, as scholars have asserted, a planing machine, a pho-nograph, or even a new weapon from World War I.[52] As a symbol of mechanized violence, however, the machine's screeching wheels and vibrating frame recall an overdetermined atmosphere of tech-nological brutality that culminated in the Great War – also known as the "war by timetable."[53] In the prewar years, the German General Staff concentrated more on improving railway effectiveness than on developing new weapons systems, and officers gained prestige for shaving minutes off of timetables.[54] By the time tensions boiled over in July 1914, a sense of railway inevitability had set in. The Ger-man military scheduled the nine railway directorates nearest the French and Russian borders to receive 530 locomotives and 8650 freight cars in just four days and envisaged sending 650 trains to France through the city of Cologne alone. Because it would take weeks for each side to transport their soldiers and weaponry to the fronts, mobilization took on the severity of a declaration of war, thus explaining Tsar Nicholas II's comical signing, then revoking, then re-signing of a general mobilization in the space of one day.[55]

His final mobilization did mean counter-mobilization and war, as illustrated by Kafka, who generally ignored the summer 1914 sabre-rattling, yet remarked on July 31: "General mobilization. K[arl] and P[epa] [Kafka's brothers-in-law] have been called up." Kafka understood first-hand that the war was a massive transporta-tion effort. He walked the next day to the crowded railway station "to see K[arl] off." The eventual declaration of war was comparatively anticlimactic, a *fait accompli* that earned only Kafka's apathy: "Germany has declared war on Russia – Swimming lessons in the afternoon" (Di 300–1).

Although military historians debate whether the intricate prewar timetabling really made war inevitable, it is clear that decades of railway planning created a material logic that overwhelmed even the General Staff. Chief of Staff von Moltke claimed on August 1, before hostilities began, that "the deployment in the West could no longer be stopped."[56] On that same day, Wilhelm II, encouraged by illusory hopes of British and French neutrality, told Moltke that Germany could concentrate its full fighting force on Russia and thus stop train movements to the West. Instead of feeling relief, Moltke insisted that structural mayhem would ensue; he became horribly distraught, suffering either a mild stroke or a nervous breakdown.[57] Timetables rendered Moltke mad just as they had done to Gregor Samsa two years earlier. Both Moltke and Samsa – likewise a military officer – know that changed plans never mean just wasting "a few hours"; rather, they catalyse a series of missed connections and possible crashes. The thought of this drives Moltke, too, "half-mad," leaving him, like Samsa, "actually unable to get out of bed" (M 10).

War timetabling also provoked unheard of rail traffic and exponentially more crashes, including the most lethal in British and French history,[58] encouraging Freud to cite the railway again in his 1920 revision of his traumatic-neurosis theory.[59] Because of the "railway disasters" and "the terrible war that has just ended," Freud sees bodies that refuse to signify anything beyond themselves (SE 18:12). They repeatedly dream of their original traumas, troubling Freud's belief in the pleasure principle and causing him to question his claim that neuroses always spring from sexual sources (see chapter 2). Unable to uncover an origin, Freud argues that these dreams might refer back to a submicroscopic injury of the cerebral cortex or the "organ of the mind," a speculation that, he realizes, embarrassingly resembles that discredited, somaticist "old, naïve theory of shock" championed by the 1880s American "railway brain" theorists and by Oppenheim (24, 31).

But Freud ventures beyond Oppenheim towards Georg Simmel's 1903 cultural criticism when he argues that the cerebral cortex develops a "shield" that protects it against the agitations of modernity, against what Simmel calls "nervous stimulation."[60] When this shield is unexpectedly breached, Freud argues, "fright" and "shock" ensue (SE 18:27, 31). As questionable as Freud's cerebral cartography is, Walter Benjamin was right to view Freud's "protective shield" as a powerful metaphor for modernity.[61] The shocks of technology increased, as did the thickness of our shields. Modern man developed a protective armour like Gregor Samsa's and, in so doing, became dialectically intertwined with the technology that he had hoped to ward off. As Max Weber argued in 1905, the very machinery that was supposed to protect and free us had become our "iron cage" (*stahlhartes Gehäuse*): in a more accurate translation, it had become a new, thicker layer of skin, our "shell as hard as steel."[62]

These theories of shields, shells, and shock give additional force to the first adjective that Kafka uses to describe Gregor's "ill" body. As we learn in the story's second sentence, Gregor is "lying on his back as hard as an armor plate [*panzerartig*]" (M 3, D 115). As Kafka would have known, *panzerartig* or *gepanzert* only became a metaphor for arthropodic exoskeletons in the eighteenth century.[63] Originally this referred to the armour that protected the medieval knight's abdomen (*Panze*) from the latest military technology of the tenth century: the tempered steel sword.[64] Similar attempts to shield the body against ever more dangerous weapons continued throughout the post-medieval era, inspiring Leonardo da Vinci's design for a set of body armour.

These technologies intensified in Kafka's day, when inventors experimented with protecting many bodies at once through armoured vehicles. Most of these trials occurred not in Germany or Britain but in Austria-Hungary. Beginning around 1900 in Pilzen, just eighty-eight kilometres from Kafka's home in Prague, a Škoda engineer patented the first "Panzerglocke": a chassis with an adjustable armoured plate. In 1906 in Vienna, Paul Daimler invented the world's first fully armoured vehicle, the "Panzerwagen." And in 1911, the year before Kafka wrote *The Metamorphosis*, the Austrian lieutenant Gunther Burstyn designed the first modern tank, complete with tractor, turret, and chain drive. Although the Austrian command rejected Burstyn's design as fantastical, his creation demonstrated how the dialectic between new weaponry and new armour climaxed – in preparation for war – just one year before Kafka invented Gregor's *panzerartigen* body.

This context connects Gregor's body to the contemporaneous theories about the brain's "protective shield" and, now more specifically, to the trauma of war. At the moment in the story when Gregor first leaves his room and exposes his grotesque body to his family, he sees something that strikes the reader initially as unimportant. Gregor spots a photograph of himself, dressed in military garb: "On the wall directly opposite hung a photograph of Gregor from his army days, in a lieutenant's uniform, his hand on his sword, a carefree smile on his lips, demanding respect for his bearing and rank" (M 17). Scholars have generally read past this image. If they mention it at all, they see it only as a reflection of Kafka's one-time fantasy of joining the army, leading to the presumption that he truly viewed this soldier as the "carefree" opposite of Gregor, the "monstrous vermin."[65] But can we really read Kafka's description on November 17, 1912 of a carefree Austrian officer with his hand on his sword unironically? More specifically, can we consider this officer to be free of the cares of actually dying at war?

World War I of course started after Kafka wrote *The Metamorphosis*, but the bloodiest confrontation on European soil since 1871 – the First Balkan War – began on October 21, just a few weeks before Kafka started his story. European armaments manufacturers used the war as a proving ground for new weapons, and the casualty counts were high. In the war's first weeks alone, the Turks lost over 100,000 soldiers while the victorious aggressors – the Serbs, Bulgarians, Greeks, and Montenegrins – lost almost 130,000. And this does not include the tens of thousands of civilians killed on both sides. The Balkan War was the first modern one to target civilians, leading to unspeakable atrocities – prefiguring the Second World War as much as the First.[66] Soldiers torched villages, butchered the faces of captured enemies, and poisoned wells. The Western press referred to the "Balkan Slaughterhouse" and documented this with brutal newspaper images, especially in neighbouring Austria-Hungary (figure 8).[67]

It is impossible to gauge the effect of the war on Kafka, because he is as reticent about it as he is about other world events. But he could not have avoided the daily headlines and appalling images in

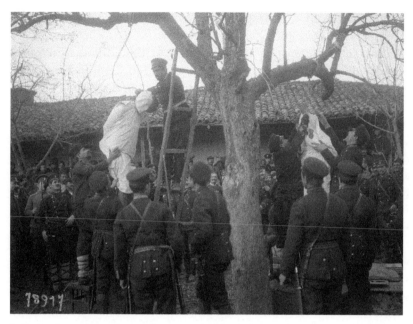

8. Bulgarian soldiers hanging two Turkish men during the First Balkan War, 1912. © Maurice-Louis Branger / Roger-Viollet.

the *Prager Tagblatt*, which he read every day, or the rumours of imminent war between Austria and Russia (through Russia's support of the Balkan League). The two great armies advanced towards their shared border in Galicia, and the Austrian navy mobilized. Already on October 27, Kafka told Felice Bauer that he was saddened by the Turkish losses – which were "a great blow to our colonies" – and he forced himself to suppress all thoughts of the war, as Hoffmann did after the Battle of Dresden: "there is nothing to do but shut one's eyes and ears and burrow into one's usual occupations" (LF 14). But even if Kafka forcibly shut his eyes, his family did not. They worried about what would happen to their asbestos factory if Kafka and his brother-in-law Karl were called up. The family even postponed the wedding of Kafka's sister, Valli.[68]

On October 30, after the beginning of the Battle of Lule Burgas, the deadliest of the entire war, Kafka lamented to Max Brod about "the misery of the Turks."[69] Two days later, Kafka told Bauer that his nightmares were dominated by images of Montenegrin soldiers, who, it was rumoured, cut off the lips and noses of captured Turks as trophies: "For a whole week I saw nothing but Montenegrins in my sleep" (LF 22).[70] Just a couple of weeks after this, on November 17, Kafka invented his *gepanzerten* hero, Gregor Samsa, and has this hero view himself in military garb. This compels us to at least consider the flip side of the traditional interpretation of this image. Just because Samsa views his previous soldier-self as "carefree" does not mean that this is true. For Samsa has misunderstood many aspects of his life, including, notoriously, the financial situation of his father. From this perspective, Samsa's vision of his soldier-life as carefree is a nostalgic fantasy, an image of himself in a state other than that of a panicked insect. In reality, a young 1912 officer in a militaristic empire who "demands" respect for his uniform is just as alienated as a travelling salesman who works day in and day out for his mendacious family. Kafka's Lieutenant Samsa thus recalls Schnitzler's alienated Lieutenant Gustl, whom Kafka would have known from the famous, eponymous 1900 satire of the Austrian military.

More than this, an Austrian officer at the brink of the Balkan Wars faced possible traumas that even a daily train-travelling salesman could not have imagined. As Erich Maria Remarque would soon report, World War I was the most brutal European war yet – especially because of the tanks, which charged "armoured" (*gepanzert*) at Remarque and his comrades. The tanks "embody for us the horror of war," Remarque writes: they roll "without feeling into the craters, ... a fleet of roaring, smoke-spewing *Panzer*, invulnerable steel beasts squashing the dead and the wounded – we shrivel up in our thin skin before them, against their colossal force our arms are pieces of straw."[71] An officer who would theoretically soon have to face such British and French tanks, Lieutenant Samsa is not the carefree opposite of insect Samsa. He is rather that strange vermin's techno-neurotic relative: its predecessor (together with the Samsa the train traveller) and its successor. Lieutenant Samsa is the soon-to-be front-soldier who will armour his "thin skin" with the latest technology – the steel helmet – yet succumb to the still thicker skin of these armoured beasts. Lieutenant Samsa and train-traveller

Samsa coincide in this technological dialectic. Their merging produces Samsa the superbug: a human with a "shell as hard as steel," a *Panzer*. Kafka imagines all this one morning in November 1912, himself so traumatized that he cannot leave his bed.

This interpretation gains traction when we consider that the first doctor to use the term "shock" to describe the illnesses of apparently uninjured but symptomatic soldiers was not the famous Charles Myers of World War I. It was Octave Laurent, a Belgian physician who observed the Balkan Wars. If the Balkan Wars were indeed a testing ground for the new French and German artillery that the two countries were about to aim at one another, then it was also a testing ground for the effects of these weapons.[72] Laurent coined the phrase "cerebro-medullary shock" to describe the soldiers' symptoms: they suffered exhaustion, tingling, twitching, paralysis, and catalepsy from being near to explosions even when not hit by them. What is significant here is not the fact that these indications match Samsa's – although most of them do – but that Laurent, like the researchers investigating train trauma before him, assumed that he needed to locate a physical cause. He examined corpses for nerve lesions and found none, so ended up hypothesizing a source. He located this in the same spot that the medics from the Napoleonic Wars had. Speeding projectiles, Laurent claimed, caused violent vibrations in the air that damaged the soldiers' inner ears.[73]

Kafka completes *The Metamorphosis* (1912) in the middle of the Balkan Wars, and he writes "In the Penal Colony" (fall 1914) and the extant text of *The Trial* (summer 1914–January 1915) at the beginning of World War I. After this, he stops writing fiction for almost two years. When Kafka starts again in the winter of 1916–17 – following what he calls "2 years of no writing" (LF 536)[74] – he no longer depicts mechanized bodies. Trains and machines rarely appear. Kafka turns almost exclusively to rural technologies. To name just a few examples relating to travel: the horses in "A Country Doctor," the ancient "bark" of the hunter Gracchus, and Klamm's sleigh in *The Castle*. In his later years, Kafka returns to the rural traffic of Raban's home neighbourhood – before Raban began his unnerving walk towards the centre of town and the station (CS 52–6). Why? Perhaps because Kafka's literary premonitions have come true. The streets of Prague, Vienna, and Berlin are now shot through with bodies that twitch nervously, as depicted in the work of Otto Dix and others.[75] With the mechanically damaged body now in public view, it no longer belongs to Kafka's nighttime fiction but to the daylight of political action.

The start of the 1914 war changed Kafka's work life immensely, because a compelling set of new victims suffering from an apparently undeniable cause temporarily bolstered the belief in the truth of trauma. If train victims were faking their nervous quivers, these new "war shakers" were certainly not, and any doctor who asserted otherwise would have seemed unpatriotic (see figure 6). Overwhelmed by the numbers of these shakers, the Austrian imperial Ministry of the Interior revised its organizational structure in 1915 to better handle the "returning warriors."[76] The ministry delegated their care to the provincial branches of the Workers' Accident Insurance Institute throughout the empire. Because Kafka was a high-ranking legal clerk at the Prague division, this meant for him a new job description and more work. He put in longer hours, processing daily roughly eighty new "war cripples" (*Kriegskrüppel*) who lined the staircase to his office before he arrived in the morning (AS 509) (figure 9).[77] In addition, Kafka, the best writer in the office, received the crucial task of making the public aware of this crisis of nervously ill veterans. He undertook the "propaganda" work of drumming up support for their care (AS 79), writing four different public pleas in 1916–17, with the first two calling for the creation of a *Volksnervenheilanstalt*, a State Hospital for the Treatment of Nervous Diseases.

The first of these appears in October 1916 in a local newspaper, just two weeks before Kafka reads "In the Penal Colony" aloud in war-torn Munich.[78] Kafka describes here vividly the shell-shocked soldiers in the same ways that he had earlier depicted characters such as Raban's "clothed body" and the victims of the "Penal Colony" apparatus:

Shortly after the outbreak of war, a strange apparition that aroused horror and compassion appeared on our cities' streets. It was a soldier returning from the front ... His body shook incessantly, as if from a terrible shiver attack ... One then also saw others, who could move forward only

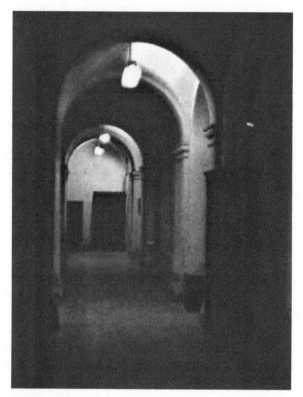

9. Hallway of the Workers' Accident Insurance Institute, where Kafka worked.
Photo: Jan Parik.

> bobbing up and down; poor, pale, emaciated men performed leaps, as if
> gripped in the back of the neck by a merciless hand that dragged them
> to and fro in these agonizing motions. (AS 494)

Like Raban's staggering "clothed body," these men signify only their
own damage, simulated or not, and seem to require scientific – not
literary – help. Yet the spare prose and sharp imagery reveal the
mixed genre of Kafka's piece. It is at once a call to arms and Kafka's
most direct contribution to the category of "war literature."[79]

As literature, it recalls Kafka's earliest fiction, the expressionist
"Description of a Struggle" (1903–7), in which characters contort

themselves in exaggeratedly painful gestures. The narrator walks with his back bent so deeply that his hands reach his knees. Then he abruptly rights himself as if being "pulled up by the hair." He later inexplicably walks zigzag in "hectic leaps." Another man flings himself on the ground, then clutches his skull "with all his strength and, moaning loudly, beat it in the palms of his hands on the stone floor" (CS 16, 27, 29).

As a call to arms, Kafka's article is an effective form of popular science, describing in laymen's term the modern neurosis doctrine created by Oppenheim and others. Kafka would have known these tenets from his work in accident insurance, and he seems to agree with them. These shaking, leaping men are suffering from "neuroses, generally traumatic ones" caused by real events (AS 494). These events also preceded the war, Kafka insists, following Oppenheim: "Slews of traumatic neuroses" appeared already in "peacetime." And the causes of these neuroses were clear: "factory accidents" (for "the working classes") and "rail transport" (for "the general population") (496–7).

A couple of weeks later, Kafka writes his second text: a public appeal for philanthropic contributions to the same *Volksnervenheilanstalt*. Here again Kafka follows Oppenheim – as Freud will four years later in *Beyond the Pleasure Principle* – this time in the social-political sense. The war is not a unique source of neuroses but part of the *longue durée* of industrial modernity. This is undoubtedly more "a war of nerves [*Krieg der Nerven*] than any earlier war," and more than this, this "nerve war" (*Nervenkrieg*) had actually already begun before 1914:

> Just as the intensive mechanization over the past decades of peace endangered the nerves of workers, leaving them deranged and ill, the monstrously increased mechanization of today's warfare has caused grave dangers and maladies to the combatants' nerves. (AS 498)

Our nervous modernity did not begin with the war, Kafka insists, and would not end with it. Unless help was found, today's iconic veteran – the "twitcher and leaper" (*Zitterer und Springer*) – would simply be added to the mass of "uncured peacetime neurasthenics,"

whose numbers would undoubtedly continue to grow after the war
(499). With these pre- and postwar victims in mind, Kafka asks for
donations from the likely culprits: the railway management as well
as the entire accident industry that springs from it – specifically, private insurance companies and social insurance institutes like the
one employing Kafka.

By viewing the war as part of a longer *Nervenkrieg* instigated by
mechanization, rapid transportation, and industrial violence, Kafka
placed the war within the context of modernity. This brought him
to concur with Oppenheim's convictions about simulation. The vast
majority of neurotics were not faking. Their symptoms had clear
material causes – industrial modernity – which had led, as Oppenheim presumed, to physical (molecular) damage. Although this
"anatomical substrate" remained submicroscopic, Kafka, like Oppenheim, seemed to be certain of its existence.[80]

The medical industry's wartime pause in the hunt for simulators
did not hold. Just two weeks before Kafka wrote the first of his public pleas, on September 21, the influential German Neurological
Society held a "War Conference" in Munich. These mainstream
neurologists concluded – in a direct attack on Oppenheim – that
the majority of war neurotics were not really ill. The doctors emphasized the cases of foreign POWs, who had experienced the same
trench warfare as the German and Austrian soldiers yet never developed neuroses – apparently because they had no fear of being sent
back to the front.[81] With the number of nervously unfit soldiers now
growing exponentially, the neurologists decided that simulation was
the greatest single crisis facing the nation. It was more dangerous
than shell shock itself. Even if the soldiers were not deliberately
faking their illness, the doctors argued, they were succumbing to
psychic fantasies: to "negative wish-ideas" (*negative Begehrungsvorstel-
lungen*) with no physical counterpart.[82]

Through this theory, the nationalist neurologists found themselves
with unlikely bed partners: the "psychogenic" camp that had gained
international momentum from the 1880s onward. Researchers such
as Charcot, Page, Janet, and Freud had long viewed neuroses as at
least partially psychic productions, a theory that the nationalist simulation hunters now used to bolster their claim that shell shock was all

in the soldiers' heads. They even employed some of Freud's terms: the "motives of illness" and the "flight into illness."[83] The simulation hunters conveniently forgot Freud's main point: that the neuroses developed unconsciously, meaning that one could speak of simulation only in a certain sense. As Freud argued as an expert witness in the postwar enquiry on military psychiatrists discussed in chapter 2, neurotics could not help but simulate. But this did not mean that they were not ill; this unconscious simulating *is* "their sickness."[84] Remarque made the same observation about "front-line madness" during the war, while watching a man try to "burrow himself into the ground with hands, feet, and mouth": "Such things are of course often simulated, but this simulating is itself a symptom [*Zeichen*]."[85] Freud agreed, but this critical position did not prevent him from enjoying psychoanalysis's sudden importance. The mainstream had indeed adopted some of his terms, and the Central Powers, he said, had "promised" in 1917 to build psychoanalytic centres behind the front (SE 17:207).

It is not clear how such centres would have jibed with the military policy of getting soldiers back to battle as quickly as possible, for as Freud noted, the long-term, "considerate, laborious and tedious" treatment essential to psychoanalysis was anathema to military necessity (SE 17:215). What is more, Freud insisted already during the war that many neurotics fled into illness with good reason ("vollberechtig") (GW 11:397). As a witness at this enquiry after the war, he claimed that military psychiatrists greatly overestimated the numbers of malingerers: "Only the smallest proportion" of soldiers were deliberate fakers (SE 17:213). Freud furthermore repudiated the military-psychiatric dogma of treating shock with more shock: erasing soldiers' "negative wish-ideas" through simulated operations, triggered choking fits, and the application of high-voltage electric currents.[86] The war neurotic's illness was "made even more intolerable to him than active service," Freud argued, compelling the man to flee "from illness into health" – and back to the front (213). This policy of making the cure worse than the disease resulted, as Freud points out, in numerous deaths and suicides.

Similarly cruel treatments, led by a certain Dr. Wiener, took place just minutes from Kafka's office. Although the average passerby did not know what went on behind these walls, Kafka would have. For he had just been made responsible for managing the "therapeutic treatment" of traumatized soldiers, especially those who were "nervously and emotionally ill" (AS 80).[87] And Kafka would have known the difference between moderate electrical therapy for neurasthenia – the same "electrification" (*Elektrisieren*) that had been prescribed for him in April 1916 – and high-voltage treatment, which was so painful as to be outlawed in parts of Germany already during the war (LF 465, BF 653).[88] Kafka would also have understood first-hand the consequences of this treatment. As an acknowledged expert on *Invalidenrenten* (pensions for war invalids), Kafka not only saw the war-shakers, he spoke and negotiated with them.[89] In his attempts to determine proper compensation, Kafka was caught up in the dilemma of simulation that divided the psychiatry community.

Even though Kafka's mechanically damaged bodies, like Gregor Samsa's, disappear from his fiction after 1914, he does not lose interest in them, at least not as a warning to himself. Six years after receiving this prescription for his own electrification, Kafka contracts a mysterious anxiety before a twelve-hour train trip to visit Oskar Baum in the German town of Georgental. After wondering aloud whether he has the widespread pathology known as "Reiseangst" – travel phobia – Kafka insists that, whatever the source of his fear, it is essentially existential and spiritual/psychic (*geistig*): a fear of change, a fear of not writing, even a fear of death. His sister Ottla disagrees, claiming that his fear's source is physical. Kafka resists her interpretation but must sense, despite his protests, that his "psychic" source is ultimately as elusive as Ottla's physical one (L 333, 336; B 384, 388). As researchers on train and war traumas – including Freud – discovered, there are symptomatic bodies that seem to have neither a detectable physical injury nor a hidden psychic one: molecular damage cannot be proven and psychic explanations "cease to carry weight" (Freud, SE 18:32). Just as Gregor's mechanized body becomes a broken sign – lacking both a clear physical injury and a psychic one stemming from his childhood – Kafka's body might also end up referring only to itself: "twitching and leaping" on the streets of Prague.

A hospital for nervous diseases like the one Kafka proposes in 1916 could symbolize hope, but this hope is as blurry as the hospital outside of Gregor's window. Neurology and psychiatry have failed to discover an original "cause," only a *mise en abyme* of submicroscopic substrata and pathological simulation. Kafka fears precisely this un-diagnosability, this etiology vaguer than tissue damage, childhood trauma, or even the "fear of death" (L 334). This unnameable inju-ry's source, as with Nordau's "degeneration," seems partially to be a nebulous cocktail of modernity: the "little shocks [*Erschütterungen*] during railway journeys," "perpetual noises," and the "continual expectation of the newspaper, of the postman." This "vertigo and whirl of our frantic life" produces rapid-fire "sensory impressions" that eventually create symptoms.[90]

The first victims of this scourge of modernity were, as Kafka knew, the weak: women and "feminine" men.[91] This fear of being labelled feminine may explain why he insisted that he was suffering *not* from the hysterical disorder of "travel anxiety" (*Reiseangst*) and *not* from what he, following Nordau, called "weakness of will" (*Willens-schwäche*) (L 333, B 384).[92] Kafka knew that physicians considered Jewish men to be predisposed to neurotic weaknesses such as rail-way hysteria, precisely because Jews were stigmatized as feminine.[93] Kafka thus understands that what happened to Gregor could hap-pen to anyone, especially to a weakened Jewish company manager (proxy, "Prokurist") like himself, who, like Gregor, has been stuck riding the rails for years. "What had happened to [Gregor] today could one day happen even to the manager [*Prokurist*]; you really had to grant the possibility" (M 10, D 125–6).[94]

This fear of an undiagnosable injury brought on by the mysteries of modernity puts a fine point on my argument. To be clear: I am not claiming that Gregor's transformation is a direct result of train trauma. Such trauma cannot cause a man to turn into a giant bug. Nor am I arguing that Gregor is a malingerer, at least not in the sense suspected by the *Kassenarzt*. Rather, I see Gregor as embodying the modern technological anxiety of indeterminacy, in which even the victims do not know whether they are ill and in which simulation itself becomes the illness. Gregor's body is modernity's prototypical broken sign: a conglomeration of symptoms that does not refer to a clear physical cause. Significant here is Kafka's decision to transform Gregor into an "Ungeziefer" (vermin), a creature "not suited for sacrifice": an un-animal existing somewhere between beast and man.[95] This uncategorizability marries Kafka's interest in medico-legal trauma to his famous "Schriftstellersein" (being-as-a-writer). For although Kafka thought deeply about trains and industrial trauma (his professional writings and diaries reveal great compassion for injured factory workers),[96] his obsession lay elsewhere. Zolaesque moments appear in Kafka's work, but such realist political exposés were never his end goal – not even on this more sophisticated level of presenting modern bodies' tragic undiagnosability. Rather, Kafka sees in trauma's semiotic dubiousness the social *condition* for his poetics – at once its catalyst and its verification.

As critics have demonstrated for decades, Kafka's writing sprang out of his "despair" of metaphor and metaphoric language: vehicles did not refer back to tenors just as signifiers did not point to signifieds (Di 398).[97] Like language itself, Gregor's body emphasizes this unreadability. This body is an accumulation of symptoms without causes and, as such, *the* cipher for Kafka's original combining of literary and medico-legal discourses. Kafka emphasizes how the *Sprachkrise* of his era was also a linguistic *trauma*, connected to the traumatized bodies around him and the ground for a poetics that truly investigates the suffering of indeterminacy. As discussed in my introduction, Kafka, like Freud, succeeds here in finding a language that is both "medical" and "literary": a language that explains traumatic suffering and gives it a voice.

Kafka had halted this project in early 1915, when he temporarily stopped writing fiction. Part of the reason was an increased workload; Kafka had to help at the family asbestos factory and eventually had to return to his office at the Accident Insurance Institute also for an evening shift, reducing his writing time.[98] But his understanding of his role as a writer in the catastrophic world around him probably also stimulated this break. The technological trauma that Kafka once only imagined had now become real. In the words of Hoffmann in Dresden one hundred years earlier: "What I have so often seen in dreams has come true – in a dreadful way – mutilated disjointed humans!!" (T 471). Gregor's train-damaged body and, more obviously, the mutilated officer from "In the Penal Colony," were now right in front of Kafka, in the staircase of his workplace. The exotic world of colonial machine torture had come to Prague: through the effects of both war and the military-psychiatric torture practised on traumatized soldiers around the corner from Kafka's office. With the technological nightmare of Kafka's fiction realized, did he still need to imagine and write stories about it? Might he have found it now more important to devote his literary energies to helping these pitiful "apparitions" that appeared before him? The masterful literary aspects of Kafka's 1916 public pleas for shell-shock victims suggest as much. His writing is here no longer just the representation of "my dreamlike inner life" but also a tool for generating compassion and social change (Di 302).

When Kafka does start writing fiction again in the winter of 1916–17, after an almost two-year hiatus, his stories famously become more parabolic, and all connections to the war seem to disappear. The editors of the only book devoted to Kafka and the First World War admit this, yet they and their contributors still try to uncover hidden "discursive" relations to the war "in the broadest sense."[99] Even if some of these attempts are revelatory, I would like to insist that, instead of searching for oblique allusions, we take Kafka's erasure of the war seriously. I see in this erasure precisely Kafka's preoccupation with the war – specifically, with the war neurotics and their relation to his struggles with literary form. My point is that Kafka's later texts engage even more intensively than *The Metamorphosis* with the same *structural* dilemma that he grappled with as an adjudicator of wartime disability claims: the unstable, possibly simulated, relation between symptom and source.

In this new fiction, Kafka deliberately heightens the causal crisis of trauma that he had exposed in *The Metamorphosis*. He describes characters who suffer from mysterious symptoms that again cannot be traced back to what Gregor Samsa calls an original "cause" (M 18). But whereas Gregor's profession and his self-diagnoses at least pointed towards a contemporaneous discourse of trauma – train travel – these late stories do not contain a hint of such a source. From the winter of 1916–17 to his death in 1924, Kafka wrote one novel and approximately fifty stories, but only one brief

tale ("First Distress") features modern technology or machinery.[100]
The meagre exceptions in the margins prove the rule. An untitled
1917 draft that Kafka chose to exclude from his collection *A Country Doctor* contains a telephone (N1 370–2). And a phone appears,
stunningly futuristically, in the horse-and-carriage village from the
novel-fragment *The Castle* (1922). As we can see in Kafka's 1917
manuscript of "The Hunter Gracchus," he has his protagonist, who
sails the world on an ancient barque, suddenly imagine telegraphs
and the railway. But Kafka immediately crosses out these references.
They thus do not appear at all in the (posthumously) published ver-
sions, even the most recent critical edition.[101] Only the manuscript,
with its cross-outs, reveals Kafka's method: he is deliberately effacing
technology from this later work. He is systematically catapulting his
characters backward, out of modernity. In this pre-industrial world,
their neurotic symptoms now appear to be fully disconnected from
"intensive mechanization."

This begs the question, If Kafka's characters' symptoms now have
no source, are these characters really even ill? Are they, as Gregor suspected about himself, "completely healthy" simulators? Or are they
simulators who are also ill, as Freud claimed – simulating "without
knowing it"?[102] And what is the literary significance of such symptoms?
Remarque uses the traditional medical term when explaining that,
among front-line soldiers, simulation "is itself a symptom [a 'sign,'
Zeichen]." Is Kafka noticing the same convergence between medical,
military, and literary discourse in this broken "sign of illness" – this
"Krankheitszeichen," the term that he also employs (CS 319, D 326)?
How might such a broken sign relate to Kafka's own writing, particularly to his scepticism about literature and signification itself?

The range and depth of Kafka's fascination with this malfunc-
tioning symptom is astounding. In the relatively brief period from
January 1917 to his death in 1924, he creates over a dozen distinct
characters who live with such broken "signs of illness." We see this
already in his first new burst of writing from early 1917, when he
was still working with injured veterans. Various characters appear
who, although transferred backward to a pre-industrial world,
show symptoms similar to those of the modern "war hysterics" who
crowded Kafka's office. The spectator in "Up in the Gallery" weeps

for no definite reason and, in the vein of a Freudian hysteric, exhibits his symptoms involuntarily, "without knowing it" (*ohne es zu wissen*) (CS 402, D 263). The narrator of "A Crossbreed" looks down at his strange pet – half kitten, half lamb – and sees tears dropping without a clear cause from the creature's huge whiskers. What is more, even the bodily source for these tears turns out to be missing. The narrator realizes that he does not know who is producing them: "Were they mine, were they the creature's?" (K 126). In "Eleven Sons," we see a man who "without being ill" displays an "impenetrable melancholy" and mysterious physical symptoms. He "staggers, especially in the twilight," likewise without cause (CS 421).

Kafka's most famous story from this period, when he was still in the midst of adjudicating settlements for war invalids, is "A Country Doctor," and it too opens with a patient presenting symptoms that appear to have no cause. The doctor is called to the bedside of a boy whose symptoms are typically neurotic: a "gaunt" look, "vacant eyes," and nervous volubility. His actions resemble those of a theatrical Charcotian hysteric, as the doctor reports: he "clings to my neck" and "whispers into my ear: 'Doctor, let me die,'" then "continues to grope toward me from the bed." The doctor immediately assumes simulation. In this supposition, he resembles the "health-insurance doctor" (*Krankenkassenarzt*) whom Gregor had feared. Just as Gregor's *Kassenarzt* always proceeded from the assumption that his patients are "healthy" (*gesund*) fakers, so does this doctor need only to "confirm" this same truth that he already knows. After summarily putting his ear to the boy's chest, the doctor decides that this boy too is perfectly "healthy" (*gesund*). He is merely nervous from too much coffee and mothering; he needs simply to be "driven out of bed with a good kick" (K 62, D 256).

When the country doctor discovers that this boy "might really be sick," he becomes concerned and then perplexed. The illness's source is, like Gregor's and the war victims', mysterious. There seems to be a "wound," but this is so surreal as to not be a wound at all. It is a pink spot on the boy's side, crawling with small white-headed creatures. The doctor can only whistle in astonishment. He realizes that he cannot help because an illness such as this submits to no normal diagnosis. What on earth could cause something that itself is so unearthly? The doctor initially offers no diagnosis at all, just a metaphor: "this blossom in your side will destroy you" (K 63).

In this use of metaphor, the medical and literary-critical discourses converge. In medical diagnostics, the symptom – the surreal "wound" – should have a source, whether internal disease or external injury. In literary criticism, the metaphoric vehicle (the wound) should point to a tenor (the "meaning" of that wound). When the work of medical diagnostics fails, as the doctor's recourse to metaphor suggests, the work of poetic hermeneutics begins. What is the tenor of this wound? Does its pink colour signify the female genitalia and the doctor's repressed desire for them, or even his guilt for subjecting his servant girl (also named Rosa, or "pink") to this desire? Or do its fantastic qualities suggest the blurring of reality and dream, or even the absurdity of existence? Or does its wormy infestation signify the inevitability of death and decay (perhaps Kafka's premonition of his tuberculosis)?

But what if the wound does not signify any of these meanings commonly cited in the secondary literature? What if it is not a classical metaphor at all but rather a marker of the breakdown of metaphoricity in both literature and in the diagnostics of trauma, which was occupying Kafka while he wrote this story? The metaphor, like the medical "sign of illness" (*Krankheitszeichen*), is divided traditionally into two parts, one on the surface and one beneath. Just as the medical symptom (the wound) traditionally pointed to a "substrate," so did the metaphor's vehicle (the wound) traditionally point to a meaning "beneath" the linguistic surface (desire, absurdity, death). In the world of trauma diagnosis that Kafka inhabited professionally, this bond between symptom and substrate had broken. Symptoms no longer connected to substrates. In the story, likewise, the vehicle is severed from any single tenor; as much as readers have tried, they have been unable to fuse this wound to a meaning.

This impossibility refers us back to Kafka's suspicion of metaphor. As critics have pointed out, it is metaphor that makes Kafka "despair of writing" (Di 398). He even goes so far as to decapitate and "literalize" it, from *The Metamorphosis* onward.[103] But we can now understand this oft-cited literary suspicion in its historical, medical-legal context. The crisis of representation essential to Kafka's poetics dovetails with the hermeneutical crisis of trauma diagnosis from his professional life.[104]

This collapse of metaphoricity in the wound of the "ill" boy is even more extreme than it was in Gregor's bug body. With Gregor, Kafka at least supplied the accoutrements of "intensive mechanization": the train. Although this mechanization could not explain the transformation of a man into an insect, the railway together with the image of Gregor as a soldier, nonetheless suggested a connection to modern trauma. Gregor indeed claims to be suffering from the "occupational ailment of the traveling salesman." For the boy in "A Country Doctor," there is no such association to industrial shock. He inhabits an anachronistically premodern world of horses, candles, and smoking wood stoves. If the source of Gregor's symptoms is ultimately unlocatable – who can know whether train-travelling *really* causes trauma? – then this problem is driven to its logical extreme with the boy. What could have produced a wound like this? Nothing. At least nothing "earthly," as the doctor senses at the end (K 65). The causal relation between symptom and substrate is undone.

Just before leaving the boy, the doctor offers him a cause for his symptoms, albeit an unconvincing one: "I, who have already been in all the sickrooms near and far, tell you: your wound is not so bad. Made with two blows of the ax at an acute angle. Many offer their sides and hardly hear the ax in the forest, let alone that it is coming nearer to them." The boy is happy: "Is that really so, or are you deluding me in my fevered state?" (K 64). Forgetting for a moment the absurdity of the diagnosis (the boy was apparently born with this wound), we may ask: Why is the boy pleased? Is it the doctor's assurance that the wound is "not so bad"? But two violent blows of an ax cannot be considered minor. The key to the boy's happiness lies rather in the odd ending of the doctor's explanation: Many people long to have this diagnosis, he says, of being hit by an ax. Why? Not because it is benign (the blows would be brutal), but because this diagnosis supplies a *physical* source for the suffering. If the ax is the source, then this wound is not merely in the boy's head; it is not merely a metaphor.

In a world filled with people who longed – like Kafka's war veterans – to prove that they were *really* ill, where so many "offer their sides" yet can "hardly hear the ax in the forest," the boy knows that he should feel lucky. "Is it really so?" He asks. The doctor reassures him: "It is really so, take a government doctor's word of honor [*das Ehrenwort eines Amtsarztes*]" (K 64, D 260). This *Amtsarzt*, unlike the earlier, cynical *Kassenarzt*, gives Kafka's patient the comforting governmental lie. We now see specifically how he is, as he stated earlier, "generous" with his patients (K 62).

Readers have often viewed "A Country Doctor" as Kafka's criticism of the medical world, and this is certainly true.[105] But Kafka is not criticizing the doctors themselves – however incompetent and secretive, however reliant on magical cures. Rather, he is revealing a structure in which the public health officer, too, is trapped. In a 1917 legal world that demanded a physical cause where none was evident, the best a "generous" doctor could do was to provide the fantasy of a "real" injury: to invent the blows of the ax. For proof of a physical source was still a requirement for compensation in European tort law. The country doctor's charitable lie thus short-circuits accusations of simulation and gives the patient causal closure. More than this, as Freud argues just three years later, an actual physical injury – if the boy had indeed suffered one – might have kept him from developing a neurosis by directing his libidinal energy towards the wound (SE 18:33).

Following the surge of creativity in early 1917, Kafka writes almost nothing for three years. He starts writing again in separate bursts in summer/fall 1920 and most of 1922, and his obsession with sourceless symptoms recurs. In "The Conscription of Troops" (1920), the presiding nobleman inexplicably has "tired eyes" and is so "weak" and "exhaust[ed]" that he requires two hands just to hold his whip. "Waves of restlessness [*Unruhe*]" run through him for no apparent reason; they present themselves physically "like the shivers of a fever," even though he has no fever (CS 439–40, N2 273). The protagonist from "The Top" (1920) likewise has incomprehensible physical indicators: he abruptly feels "nauseated" and begins to wobble and "totter like a top" (CS 444). Mrs. Brunswick from Kafka's last attempt at a novel, *The Castle* (1922), resembles both these characters and Gregor Samsa. She exhibits baffling symptoms – is strikingly "pale," "infirm," and unable to speak to anyone. If she does happen to speak, she is so weakened that she must spend "days in bed" recovering. Nobody understands her illness, especially because it "wasn't actually an illness." And the source of the non-illness remains enigmatic. Although Mrs. Brunswick claims to be "fully aware of the cause of her condition," she can only "hint" at this to others. The protagonist, K., indeed doubts whether the "causes of the illness" are so clear after all. The only thing that he, and we, can know for sure is that they are slippery and undefinable: they are "fickle."[106]

Just after Kafka stopped working on *The Castle*, he wrote "The Married Couple," in which the husband suffers from similarly inexplicable symptoms. He suddenly begins "trembling" (*zitternd*) and having difficulty breathing. For no apparent reason, he finds himself bent sharply forward "as if someone were gripping or striking the back of his neck" (*als hielte oder schlüge ihn jemand im Nacken*) (CS 454, N2 539). This position recalls Kafka's 1916 newspaper plea for the *Kriegszitterer*, who likewise moved "as if they were gripped in the back of the neck by a merciless hand" (*als halte sie eine unbarmherzige Hand im Genick*) (see figure 6). Is this husband from Kafka's 1922 story a shell-shock victim in disguise? A concealed literary relative of a contemporaneous "husband" – from Hugo von Hofmannsthal's *Der Schwierige*, who, as discussed in chapter 2, exhibited in 1921 traumatic symptoms from the war? At first glance, Kafka's description suggests as much: While bent over so violently, the husband's eyes "bulge," his jaw hangs down "helplessly," and his whole face goes "out of joint." He then passes out, like a war hysteric, falling "lifeless" back into his chair. But two key differences pertain: Hofmannsthal's husband is explicitly suffering from war trauma while Kafka's is not, and Kafka brings the problem of simulation to the fore. For immediately after passing out, the husband opens his eyes, claiming to have fallen asleep simply out of boredom. And he shows no more signs of illness (CS 454–5).

In Kafka's final spurt of writing, in 1923–4, similar cases of symptoms without origins abound. His autumn 1923 story "A Little Woman," often dismissed as a biographical send-up of Kafka's landlady,[107] is actually a sophisticated depiction of the simulation quandary. The titular protagonist wakes every morning "pale," "unslept," and "oppressed by headache." In a repetition of Gregor Samsa's words, she is "unable to work." She is also prone to faintness and "tears of rage and despair." Like the husband from "The Married Couple," she exhibits the "trembling" (*Erzittern*) reminiscent of the railway and war hysterics (CS 318, 322, 321; D 328). Her family consults to and fro about "the causes" (*Ursachen*) of her condition but has "not yet found them." According to her neighbour, the story's male narrator, she thinks that *he* is the cause, but he dismisses this theory. Taking on the role of an *Amtsarzt*, he observes each of her symptoms and ultimately decides that they are only a "pretense" to "draw public attention." Knowing that "women faint easily," he concludes: "I don't much believe in these symptoms of illness [*Krankheitszeichen*]" (CS 318, 322, 319; D 324, 326).

But even if she is only simulating these *Krankheits-Zeichen*, she might still be ill. As Freud had claimed just three years earlier, the desire to simulate was itself an ailment. Mainstream neurologists refused to consider simulation unconscious and thus a sickness, but they did acknowledge that it functioned like one: it was apparently infectious, as discussed in chapter 2. The narrator of "A Little Woman" indeed finds himself now suffering, like the woman, from "Nervosität" (nervousness), which he insists he has contracted from her. She has transferred this to him by creating in his life a series of light but steady "Erschütterungen": the same word that both Freud and Nordau used to describe the continual "shaking" and "shocks" produced by the railway. The narrator attempts to fend off this nervousness by remaining "calm" (*ruhig*), but he says that she undermines this calmness through her agitation. He too now becomes "uneasy" or "un-calm" (*unruhig*) – another word that Kafka borrows here from Gregor. The narrator now repeats this word nervously, using it three times in two sentences: once as "beunruhigen" and twice as "unruhig" (CS 322, 323; D 330, 332).

The little woman infects him with her uneasiness, he claims, but this contagion becomes more complex when we remember that, at the beginning of the story, *she* had thought that he was infecting her. Both characters somehow contaminate the other. In this, the narrator confirms mainstream neurology's claim that hysteria was circular. It jumped from psyche to psyche, and one could, tragically, not pin down its origin.

The mole-like protagonist of the next story Kafka wrote, "The Burrow" (December 1923), likewise exhibits nervous, traumatic symptoms that have no clear source. This creature is paranoid, obsessive, compulsive, delusional, cries in his sleep, and is permanently anxious and unnerved. Kafka describes him, like Gregor and many of the post-1916 protagonists, as "ängstlich" (anxious) and, at least seven times, as "unruhig/beunruhigt" (agitated, unsettled, restive). The creature's constant state of "nervous anxiety" intensifies precisely because he is unable to locate the cause. He imagines a panoply of invisible enemies trying to dig their way into his burrow, but he has never seen any of them and wonders whether they even exist. The creature goes even further, doubting whether his anxieties are caused by any identifiable "outside" source at all (K 174).

Yet he nonetheless continues his quest for external sources, focusing now on a faint sound, so quiet that the creature wonders whether he even hears it at all. But this does not stop him from hypothesizing about its cause. Does it emanate from the "small fry" whom he normally eats? Or from "unknown creatures, a migrating herd"? If yes, then why does he never manage to see any of them? He is at a loss: "What was I dealing with?" and "What was it, then?" Is it perhaps "a nothing"? Panicked about this inability to find the noisemaker that should be the source of his neurasthenia, the creature frantically drags his ear along the walls of his burrow and even "tears open the soil" – yet still does not find anything (K 179, 181, 182).

Recent scholars have pointed to a possible source of the creature's neurosis by connecting it to trauma in World War I. The "trenches" (*Graben*) in Kafka's burrow indeed remind us of Kafka's own 1915 visit to a replica trench and his work with war veterans (Di 351; figure 10).[108] More specifically, Julia Encke links the creature's frantic search for a nearly inaudible noise to soldiers listening nervously on the floors of their trenches for enemies tunnelling below. World War I soldiers in fact systematically heeded every slight sound of "hammering and knocking," which suggested digging underneath or alongside.[109] Kafka's creature likewise dreads even "innocent" sounds, pressing his ear against the wall and "listening attentively" to every murmur. He constructs a "trial trench" (*Versuchsgraben*) in order pre-emptively to eradicate this burrowing "enemy" (K 177, 171, 172; N2 594).

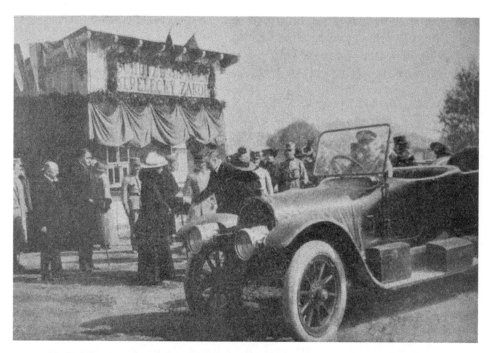

10. Entrance to the replica trench in Prague, which Kafka visited in 1915.
From Stach, *Kafka: Die Jahre der Erkenntnis.*

In the war, the enemy was generally attempting to lay mines that
would collapse the opposing trench and bury the soldiers alive –
sometimes tens of thousands at once, as in the 1917 Battle of Messines. Trench soldiers lived in constant fear of such a burial, and
Kafka's creature dreads this too. He fears "suffocation" and, more
than this, considers ways of "suffocating" his enemy within the burrow (K 176, 168). Ultimately, he contemplates using this specific war
tactic of burying his enemy alive. He will collapse his own trench
through an "Erdverschüttung," he says, employing the term which
delineated, during the war, the manoeuvre of burying the enemy
beneath "a fall of earth" (N2 625).[110] In Freud's 1920 memorandum
for an enquiry on psychiatrists' brutal treatment of soldiers, he indeed names "Erdverschüttung" as one of the two primary sources
of trauma during the war (see chapter 2). When Kafka's creature

considers deploying an *Erdverschüttung,* he furthers his earlier fantasy of suffocating his enemy. He will "bury" him and in so doing either kill or severely traumatize him, thereby preventing this enemy from using the same tactic against him (K 187).

As compelling as such a reading is, it leaves open the question of why Kafka seems to confound this – and any – attempt to locate a source for the creature's neurasthenia. First, as in most of his post-1916 writings, Kafka constructs a premodern world that rigorously excludes both the war and any contemporaneous technology; we see no relation between the creature's hysteria and industrialization. Kafka even avoids metaphors borrowed from modern technology. The protagonist fears that the enemy beast, for example, is "boring/drilling" (*bohren*) his sharp snout into the burrow, but Kafka limits this boring to the animal's snout, never comparing it to a mechanical bore, even though the handheld electric drill (*Bohrmaschine*) was invented during Kafka's childhood. Second and most important, Kafka repeatedly undermines any relation between symptom and cause within the text, which hints at his larger poetics of indeterminacy, in which – as in *The Metamorphosis* – the hero's body cannot be read as a metaphor for something else. Just as the creature cannot locate a source of his neurasthenia outside of his body or outside of the world of his burrow, Kafka's readers cannot locate a meaning for these symptoms outside of the text itself.

The creature senses that the source of his worries is indeed not "outside" at all but inside: "weit zurückgedrängt" – in Corngold's rendering, "deeply repressed." This translation implies a psychoanalytic surface-depth model, with the creature's anxious symptoms pointing to a hidden internal truth. But the phrase's actual nonclinical meaning – "pushed far back" – together with its syntactical context suggests something different. As the creature insists, the effects of his internal "pushed-far-back" worries are exactly "the same as those of the worries that life outside produces" (K 174, N2 600). Outside and inside are identical, he claims. We do not here have the Freudian model of repression, which is structured on difference: the internal truth appears disguised as the external symptom, which we need to decode.

We see this same collapsing of the difference between outside and inside later, after the creature tears through the walls of his burrow and finds nothing. He senses that his symptoms of nervousness or disquiet ("Unruhe") point to something internal but again not in the sense of a distorted corporeal symptom pointing towards a deep coded truth. Rather, in Kafka's world, this symptom of trauma – the physical *Unruhe* of scratching at walls – points only to itself. The creature continues to tear at the walls now not in order to find something "but to do something that matches [his] inner disquiet [*Unruhe*]" (K 182, N2 615). He produces an external activity that corresponds to an internal feeling: external *Unruhe* is "the same" as internal *Unruhe*. In semiotic terms, there is no longer a relation between signifier and signified – only an equivalence. The sign is more than just broken. There is no sign at all, no semiotic relation. *Unruhe* points only to *Unruhe*. Just as Gregor Samsa's body signified not train trauma but rather a discourse of trauma in which the sign itself was shattered, so too does the creature's trauma point not to the war but to the diagnostic crisis of the war, in which the physical symptom was tragically unable to point to the event that caused it. The creature's body, like so many traumatized bodies of his day, could refer only to itself.

The final prominent example of this simulation crisis appears in Kafka's last story, the 1924 "Josefine, the Singer or The Mouse People," where the protagonist suffers from a general "nervous discontent" and telltale hysterical symptoms. Her voice is "strained" and almost inaudible; she has fits of foot-stamping, swearing, and biting; and her body "vibrat[es] in a terrifying way" – recalling those who suffered mechanical violence in wars and train travel (K 100, 97). Even more directly than Kafka's other stories, "Josefine" combines the problem of simulation with Kafka's job adjudicating accident insurance claims before, during, and after the war. Like Gregor and the "little woman," Josefine says towards the end of the story that her symptoms render her incapable of working. The story's narrator repeats here exactly the diction of Gregor's "insurance doctor" when he asks himself whether Josefine is shirking: How could she possibly be "work shy" (*arbeitsscheu*), he wonders, when this syndrome is completely unknown among the mouse people? And he reports on her recurring petitions to be, like the injured who appeared in Kafka's office, "excused from all work" (K 104, D 370).

The narrator describes Josefine's case in the specific language of the postwar insurance crisis. Just as war veterans, like the injured factory workers before them, engaged in a well-known legal *Renten-kampf* – a "fight" or "struggle" for their pensions that often dragged through the courts for years – Josefine engages in a long-term "strug-gle" to be excused from work.[111] The narrator uses this term from the pension battles – *Kampf* or *kämpfen* – to describe Josefine's fight for a "work exemption" at least eleven times in just four pages, a fact obscured in English translations that mitigate repetition through synonyms. The Muirs use "struggle," "fight," "pursue," "attack," "battle," and "campaign." In one crucial paragraph, for example, they shift between "battle," "campaign," and "fight." Josefine has:

> transferred the battle [*Kampf*] for her rights from the field of song to another which she cares little about ... When it comes to her campaign [*Kampf*] for exemption from work, we get a different story; it is of course also a campaign [*Kampf*] on behalf of her singing, yet she is not fight-ing [*kämpft*] directly with the priceless weapon of her song. (CS 374, D 372–3)

Corngold remains more loyal to *Kampf,* alternating in these eleven usages only between "struggle" and "fight," but he does still alter-nate – as we see in this same passage. Josefine has:

> shifted the struggle [*Kampf*] for her rights from the domain of song to another area, one that means less to her ... It is another matter, however, with her struggle [*Kampf*] to be excused from work; true, this struggle [*Kampf*] also concerns her song, but here she is not fighting [*kämpft*] directly with the precious weapon of her song. (K 105–6)

The most literal translation would insist on Kafka's deliberate repetition of *Kampf,* rendering the key passage: "It is another mat-ter, however, with her struggle to be excused from work; true, this struggle also concerns her song, but here she is not struggling ..."

And this repetition would have to be given consistently through-out: Josefine has, for a long time, "struggled … to be excused from all work." Year after year, she "takes up the struggle," even though no one "finds this struggle amusing." She "does not allow them to frighten her off the struggle. Lately the struggle has grown even more critical." Josefine refuses to back down from this "struggle for an *Arbeitsbefreiung* [the legal term in Kafka's day for an official ex-emption from work]" (D 368, 369, 370, 372, 373).

Kafka matches this repetition of "Kampf" with that of "Forderung," which denotes "demand" but more specifically a "claim" or "pe-tition" made by someone in a legal struggle. Kafka uses *Forderung* ten times in these same four pages to describe Josefine's petition to be exempted from a work; this repetition is again obscured in translation. The Muirs vary between "demand" and "petition," and Corngold between "claim" and "demand." But Kafka insists on the repetition of the single word, *Forderung*. A strict rendering of some of these passages reveals the same effect of recurrence: "It is with this petition that [Josefine] will stand or fall" despite the commu-nity's "treatment of Josefine's petition"; one could argue, "from the mere oddness of this petition, from the spiritual attitude needed to think up such a petition, that it has an inner justification. But our people draw other conclusions and calmly reject the petition" (D 370, 373, 369).[112] Kafka's lexical reiterations are stylistically in-felicitous, so there must be a reason why he employs them. And this reason could well be Josefine's resemblance to the complain-ants who appeared in his office. Josefine makes a "petition" in the "struggle" for her pension, and she will not desist until she receives a legal "decision" – *Entscheidung*, denoting also "adjudication" – in her favour (K 106, D 374). This was the type of adjudication for which Kafka was responsible. At its crux lies the crisis of simulation.

Josefine's struggle for her pension is also a struggle against her "people" (*Volk*). As such, it performs the social conflict at the heart of all forms of insurance. Insurance spreads risks from individuals to a larger community, and in so doing, creates tension between that community and the individual. The narrator sees this in Josefine's struggle and, like the narrator in "A Little Woman," reveals sympa-thies with the community. Josefine, the narrator writes, "expects to be relieved of all the cares of earning her daily bread and everything connected with our struggle for existence and – presumably – shift the burden to the whole populace" (K 104). When the people decide that Josefine is not truly injured, they choose to reject her petition. In so doing, they act as a decision-making indemnificatory body, a corporation of insurance. They decide not to bear the responsibility for her individual subsistence.

The narrator, now employing the first-person plural, says that "we" do not feel good about this – for each member of the community now realizes that he could be next. "He" could feel the community's coldness just as Josefine had: "the people [*Volk*] might at some time behave toward him in a similar way" (K 104–5). Like the welfare state that Bismarck's Germany began implementing in the year Kafka was born, Josefine's *Volk* regards itself as parental – feeling "fatherly concern" for each individual. This *Volk* is the *Vater Staat* (father-state) that soon appeared too in Austria-Hungary. Yet this paternal community is also capable of cutting itself off "inscrutably from a comrade" and leaving one of its own mercilessly in the lurch (105). Each individual knows that this fate could be hers or his. This reveals the fragility of every individual's position in relation to the community. This tension appears stylistically in the narrator's many switches from the first-person plural to the first-person singular, from the voice of the insuring group to that of the endangered individual – beginning already on the first page: "*Our* [*Unsere*] singer is named Josefine," yet "*I* [*Ich*] have often considered ..." (K 94–5, D 350).

The crisis of simulation and insurance comes here to the fore. Having had her petition refused so many times, Josefine now presents a dramatic physical injury to the community, claiming that it interferes with her ability to entertain them. She resembles a pension petitioner in Kafka's office or even Kafka himself, whose illnesses often got him exemptions from his office job. She claims that she has "hurt her foot at work." She can no longer stand for long periods, she claims, and because she can only sing while standing, her songs will have to be foreshortened. To dramatize her injury, she "limps and leans on her followers," lets herself "be led around like a cripple," and shows herself in her "pitiful condition more often than usual" (K 106).

The narrator adopts again the position of the community and restates the problem of insurance. The community must assess whether the individual is truly injured before granting benefits. Otherwise everyone could, like Gregor Samsa and the "little woman," declare himself unable to work. If each of us limped as dramatically as Josefine does "every time we suffered a scrape," the narrator pronounces, there would "be no end to the entire people's limping." The community now hardens its initial position against Josefine. They decide conclusively that she is simulating: "No one believes that her injury is real" (K 106).

This brings Josefine to her final tactic. Like many of the hysterics treated by Freud and the war neurotics assessed by Kafka, she no longer claims even to have a physical injury but rather an all-encompassing, indeterminate malaise. She uses some of the same terms popular in the hysteria diagnoses of the day. Her complaints now are of "Müdigkeit" (fatigue), "Schwäche" (feeling faint or weak), and the fin-de-siècle catch-all for ill humours: "Mißstimmung" (dysphoria or bad mood). Her entourage must beg and implore her, in vain, to at least try to sing. They carry her limp body to her spot on the stage. The narrator, speaking for the community, has had enough: "So now, in addition to a concert, we have a theatrical play [*Schauspiel*]." This charade ends with her, like so many late Kafka characters, bursting into "inexplicable tears" (*undeutbaren Tränen*) and then, at the point when she tries to sing, "collapsing before our eyes." As if to reinforce the suspicion of simulation, the narrator announces that Josefine suddenly becomes, like the husband in "The Married Couple," healthy again. She sings with unusual feeling and then trots off the stage powerfully, with "a firm gait," miraculously not needing any help and instead glaring coldly at her sceptical audience (K 107, D 375).

In the story's epilogue, Josefine disappears, and the narrator, speaking again in the plural voice of the community, explains that Josefine has "abandoned us" out of revenge. But this abandoning only reveals how little Josefine understands "us," as well as the nature of an insurance community. The narrator employs the diction of accounting to explain her misperceptions: "Strange how badly she calculates, our clever Josefine, so badly that you have to think she doesn't calculate at all." Her false calculations emanate from a misunderstanding about insurance's communal body. This body either offers "fatherly concern" or it does not, based on a judgment of truth or simulation. But it does not have an emotional relation to the individual, even though "we" still prefer to use the paternal metaphor. For this reason, when Josefine disappears, "our" people remain "calm" and "imperious," "showing no disappointment" – remaining "an immovable body" of insurance that simply "continues on its way" (K 107).

Josefine has furthermore misunderstood the community's relation to her emotional "gift," her singing. Just as the community is unaffected by her departure, so too were they never dependent on her art. Her people are indeed "an immovable body," which, "despite appearances to the contrary, can only bestow gifts and never receive them" (K 107). Like the Bismarckian state, which invented Kafka's profession of accident insurance and served as a model for Austria-Hungary's version, Josefine's community does not rue the loss of her singing. Despite appearances, her people never really needed this. When it comes to gifts like this, the community can only bestow and, furthermore, can only bestow one specific gift: social security. In return, it demands no gifts and certainly not aesthetic ones. It demands only work and – essential to this – an agreement not to simulate.

Whoever breaks this agreement is, like Josefine, refused the gift of communal sanctuary. The community does not weep after losing Josefine. It simply "continues on its way." And because this is the way of insurance, it insists not on a process of mourning but on a recalculation. The headcount must be readjusted. As we learn in the story's final sentence, Josefine, the shunned simulator, is subtracted from the number of insurable bodies. But she is more than just subtracted. She is removed from the very idea of calculation: she becomes "incalculable" (*zahllos*). She has now joined an "incalculable mass" that lives outside of the insurance community, whether because of death or departure (K 108, D 377). This number is *zahllos* – literally, "without a number." For the insurance community needs numbers only for those inside of it. The vast seas of people on the outside require no counting.

The narrator closes by saying that, because "we practice no history," we will not only cease to count Josefine; we will also forget her (K 108). But can he, or his brethren, really forget the drama of social security that Josefine performed? Is not his story itself a record of how it cannot be forgotten? The narrator's labile shifts from the "we" to the "I" give perfect aesthetic form to the pertinence of Josefine's story for the community. Each individual knows that she could be next. She, too, could move from the secure plural to the exiled singular. She, too, could become the person who claims to be ill but finds no relation between her *Krankheitszeichen* – her signs of illness, her symptoms – and an underlying physical lesion. Like the insurance industry of Kafka's day, Josefine's community insists on a pathological physical substrate. General "dysphoria" does not suffice. And simulation remains the enemy of the people. Only once do the people imagine, as Freud does, that someone could be simulating *and* sick – that the very desire to simulate could be the marker of illness: Is someone like Josefine, who is "mental[ly]" capable of such a transparent performance, not, by virtue of this very capacity, actually sick and therefore "justified"? But the people ultimately reject this thought, whose ramifications explode the logic of the insurance community: "We draw different conclusions and calmly reject" her petition (K 104). The subject's tears thus remain, for the community, *undeutbar* – inexplicable. They are markers of a simulation that the community can neither understand nor abide.

As with my reading of *The Metamorphosis*, my interpretation of "Josefine" and the other late stories does not aim to solve them – especially not by definitively diagnosing their characters. To maintain that Josefine, for example, embodies the fin-de-siècle hysterical woman in conflict with the insurance industry is no more valid than insisting that she stands for the Jewish artist, Kafka's dream of a "minor literature," or his scepticism about art's role in society.[113] Such a claim would ignore the narrator's insistence that Josefine's tears, like her wheezy piping and the "clothed body's" stumblings before her, are ultimately "undeutbar," meaning "inexplicable" but implying also "uninterpretable" – recalling the popular story, "Inexplicable," that mystified Freud during the war. This *Undeutbarkeit* is central to Kafka's aesthetic, beginning already with *Wedding Preparations*, where we learn that the initial symptom of Raban's "clothed body" – its "staggering" – "indicate[s] not fear but its nothingness." Its "stumbl[ing]," Raban continues, is not "a sign of agitation [*Aufregung*]." Raban insists here that each symptom (*Krankheits-Zeichen*) is defined negatively, as what it does *not* signify. It is not capable of "indicating": it "zeigt ... nicht" (CS 55, N1 17–18). As I pointed out earlier in this chapter, this problem of broken signification extends into *The Metamorphosis*, where critics have long viewed Gregor Samsa's body as an "opaque sign" and a "free-floating" signifier.[114] This *Undeutbarkeit* continues even more powerfully, as I am arguing here, into the late stories.

While not "solving" the stories, contextualization does allow us to see Kafka's aesthetic of *Undeutbarkeit* in a new light: as a reaction to the contemporaneous attempts to find a definitive material source for the "nervous" scourge of modernity.[115] Although Kafka cites such a source in his 1916 public pleas for donations ("intensive mechanization" and the "war"), he consistently resists this in his fiction. We see this already in *Wedding Preparations* and *The Metamorphosis*, where Kafka hints initially at the possibility of railway hysteria only to subvert this diagnosis through overdetermination, hyperbole, and irony. He undermines such diagnoses more powerfully in the post-1916 stories, where readers have long noticed an increase in *Undeutbarkeit* but not the context of this increase: Kafka's wartime work at Prague's Accident Insurance Institute, where the crisis of the opaque body confronted him every day. In these stories, symptoms similar to those from the earlier work persist, but they are now fully decapitated from a source. With the exception of "First Distress" (1922), Kafka rigorously excludes modern machinery from these stories. The symptoms survive alone. Like the "little woman," Kafka's protagonists exhibit *Krankheits-Zeichen* that point to everything and nothing. These opaque signs – signifiers without apparent signifieds – disrupt the causality at the heart of contemporaneous trauma research. Their brokenness expresses the quandary of simulation.

The Poetics of Trauma: Simulation, Causality, and the Crisis of Insurance

Already in the Napoleonic Wars, as discussed in chapter 1, doctors insisted that soldiers who left the battlefield shaking and sobbing must have hidden physical injuries. Otherwise why would apparently unscathed men like Pierre Bezukhov from *War and Peace* be so mysteriously afflicted? And why would E.T.A. Hoffmann need to work through his war experience years later, as he did in "The Sandman"? Shells had flown nearby, yes, but had not hit them. The "wind of the cannonball," these physicians speculated, must have damaged the men's inner ears and sense of equilibrium. For if this were not true (as turned out to be the case), were these men even really ill?

By the first decade of the twentieth century, Kafka understood this problem well from his work in accident insurance. Nineteenth-century industrialization had produced widespread rail transport and factory accidents and, with this, swaths of "peacetime neurasthenics." Like the earlier victims from Borodino, Austerlitz, and Dresden, these men displayed neurotic symptoms but no physical injuries. Insurance industry doctors argued that they were faking. But others insisted that there must be concealed physical lesions, and they postulated injuries to the spinal column and, later, molecular damage to the brain. During the Balkan Wars, which Kafka followed in the newspapers while writing *The Metamorphosis*, the physician Octave Laurent first used the term "shock" to describe war trauma, and he, like his forerunners, searched for a somatic source. He concluded that these shaking, weeping, confused men were not faking but had, like their predecessors in the Napoleonic Wars, suffered submicro-scopic damage to their inner ears. Kafka followed these discussions about physical injury and simulation closely, even more so during World War I. He now assumed professional responsibility for the compensation of injured returning soldiers, especially the "nerv-ously and emotionally ill" ones. The question of whether a soldier was simulating thus moved to the heart of Kafka's job. At the same time, he began creating literary characters who, even more ada-mantly than Gregor Samsa, insisted that they were ill but – like the war and railway neurotics – were unable to prove this or pinpoint a physical cause.

Central to the simulation quandary was always this problem of the "pathological-anatomical substrate," not least because, as discussed in the previous chapter, the compensations that Kafka administered were impossible without it (and remained so until European law changed in the 1960s). Oppenheim and others thus argued for this substrate's presence – if only at the molecular level – even though they readily admitted that it was "undetectable."[1] Freud too, despite his insistence on the psychogenesis of neuroses, never surrendered his belief in a material source – especially after witnessing the traumas of the war (see chapter 2). After being unable to locate a convincing psychic origin for many cases of shell shock, he conceded in 1920 that when the "strength of a trauma exceeds a certain limit," psychic causes "will no doubt cease to carry weight" (SE 18:32). The traumatic neuroses present here a similar problem to what Freud had earlier called the "actual neuroses." Seemingly produced by direct physical ("toxic") damage, they stubbornly offered psychoanalysis "no points of attack"; they had to be left to "biologico-medical research" (16:389).

When there is "no doubt" of biology's primacy, trauma patients become untreatable through classical psychoanalysis. Perhaps for this reason, Freud loses interest in the traumatic neuroses after 1920. He returns to them briefly at the end of his life but then only to mention their imperviousness to therapy. As he confesses in his posthumous *Outline of Psychoanalysis*, traumatic neuroses caused by "somatic shocks" from the war and the railway ultimately repudi-ate the general rule of analysis: "their relations to determinants in childhood have hitherto eluded investigation" (SE 23:184).

But even if Freud still imagines a biological source, he, like Kafka's characters, cannot specify it. We "know nothing" about how this apparently somatic injury develops into a neurosis, Freud says, because this biological/chemical trajectory is hidden within the "excitatory process that takes place in the elements of the psychical systems." We are, Freud concludes, "consequently operating with a large unknown factor" – literally, "with a big X" (*mit einem großen X*). Freud's "big X" deftly expresses the two major knots in the history of trauma that persist to our present day. The first is the same one Nordau had tried to untangle in *Degeneration*: What precisely is modernity's effect on the "organ of the mind" (Freud, SE 18:30–1, GW 13:31)? The second is: Even if we can attribute some specific degenerative cerebral effects to industrialization and war, how do we connect these to neurotic symptoms?

This second knot is especially gnarled because the traumatic neuroses speak specifically to the man who was *not* hit by the shell or injured in the train. Does such a near miss even produce the mysterious cerebral "toxicity" or "lesion" sought by fin-de-siècle neurologists? And even now, when neurologists have the endocrinological and imaging capacities of which Freud only dreamt, this problem of connecting hormones or lesions to symptoms persists. The DSM-5 defines post-traumatic stress disorder (PTSD) as a "trauma- and stressor-related disorder" that generally lacks an identifiable somatic injury. Brain injuries have indeed not been found in the majority of today's PTSD sufferers; likewise, most soldiers who suffer brain injuries do not develop PTSD.[2] Although some scientists argue that all PTSD symptoms must have a biological counterpart, they too waver on whether these biological changes are the cause or the effect of the symptoms (see chapter 2). The larger debate about the existence of somatic etiology thus still pertains, thrusting us back to the same etiological question that confronted Freud and his contemporaries a century ago: When a shell lands in a trench next to two men, why does only one of them develop traumatic symptoms? Might the causal problem itself be so complex that we can never find a straightforward biological source? Might every symptom ultimately have so many causes that the etiological discussion becomes absurd?

Many physicians at the fin de siècle confronted this problem by extending the term "cause" to something more like "condition." *M. tuberculosis*, for example, was a necessary but not "unique or sufficient" cause of tubercular disease – remaining latent in the vast majority of people (Kafka being among the minority of carriers to actually contract the illness).[3] Many other factors such as malnourishment, overcrowding, and smoking determined whether the bacteria produced symptoms. We are experiencing a similar causal conundrum today: you can carry the virus SARS-CoV-2 without becoming ill with Covid-19. The same enigma pertained for hysteria. A railway accident, an enemy shell, or being buried alive in a trench did not necessarily create symptoms. You were more likely to experience these if, as Nordau argued, you were an alcoholic or suffered from "weakness of will."[4] Freud and many others adopted the wide-ranging term "predisposition" to encompass these contributing causes. For Freud, people with insufficiently "cathected" psychic systems, often due to neurotic fantasies from childhood, were more likely to become neurotically ill.

Even though most of today's psychiatrists disagree with Freud's theory of inadequate cathexis, they are still trying to solve this same mystery of etiology – as we see in today's medical insurance debates about "pre-existing conditions." The problem then, as now, was not that there was no cause but that there were too many. As discussed in my introduction: overdetermination coincides here with indeterminacy. And even in the rare cases where there is evidence of a remarkable physical lesion – as after a shelling or a railway accident – the relation of this "source" to the symptom remains mysterious, an ultimately unknowable "big X."

This tension between material and psychic sources, and between sources and symptoms, plays itself out on Kafka's own body just three years after Freud described the "big X." In July 1922, as discussed in chapter 3, Oskar Baum invited Kafka to visit him in Georgental. Kafka initially agrees to go, but then he, like Josefine, suffers a breakdown. He stays awake all night, seeming at first to have contracted what he calls a bad case of travel phobia ("Reiseangst"). Kafka's sister, Ottla, insists that this phobia's source is primarily "physical," suggesting that the tubercular Kafka has good reason to fear a twelve-hour journey. Contemporary researchers in fact argued that train travel could worsen existing tuberculosis and even catalyse "tubercular processes" in the healthy (as well as infect fellow travellers).[5] What is more, many contended – following Oppenheim and Nordau – that train-induced damage to the brain and nervous system could result in breakdowns, like the one that Kafka had just had. Kafka is only partially joking when he asks Baum whether he might be able to complete this long train trip instead on a series of streetcars.[6]

As if warning himself not to board this train, Kafka creates a story in this same 1922 summer that brings modern machinery back to the forefront of his writing for the first (and last) time since 1914. The protagonist of "First Distress," like Gregor Samsa, insists that his constant journeying, especially in the "railway train" (*Eisenbahnzug*), is "zerstörend" – destructive, wrecking, ruinous – to his "nerves." This first Kafka character to board any sort of modern vehicle in almost a decade now displays the same nervous symptoms experienced by the characters from *Wedding Preparations* through to the late stories: he "shudders," "bursts into tears," and "sobs" (K 85, 86; D 319). Yet only now, because of Kafka's looming train trip to Georgental, does this dubious technological source from the early stories reappear.

As in Kafka's earlier stories, the primacy of this mechanical basis immediately gives way, in "First Distress," to a psychological one. The protagonist seems mostly to be suffering from "thoughts" that obsess him (K 86). Kafka, likewise, when fretting over the trip to Georgental, denies that his phobia is as simple as a fear of travel: "It is not *Reiseangst*." He insists that his condition is mostly "psychic" and that this mental source itself is inscrutably diffuse, splitting into a dazzling series of fears: "fear of change," "fear of attracting the attention of the gods," "fear of death," "fear ... that I will be kept away from the desk for at least several days," and finally "fear in general" (L 333, 335, 338).

These abstractions seem on the one hand to be disavowals of something that Kafka senses to be true. As discussed in chapter 3, the just-pensioned Kafka fears that he, like the protagonists of "First Distress," "Josefine, the Singer," and "A Little Woman," is physically weak, feminine, and hysterical. And all of this manifested itself as a pathological fear of trains, a "railway phobia" (*Eisenbahnphobie*) like the one that had paralysed Freud twenty-five years earlier (see chapter 2). So, Kafka gets defensive, insisting that there is nothing wrong with him. He protests too much, like the neurotic narrators of "Researches of a Dog" and "A Little Woman": "I was at my full strength and in perfect health"; "I shall quietly continue to live my own life for a long time to come, untroubled by the world" (K 154, CS 324). Kafka too claims that he is perfectly fine. His fears are, first, not physical but psychic and, now, not psychic but existential – common to every man. He is not hysterical, merely cursed by the gods (L 333). On the other hand, he ultimately lets this resistance subside, allowing all possible diagnoses. Unlike Freud, who concealed his railway phobia,[7] Kafka trumpets this possibility to five different people in one week: Ottla, Baum, Max Brod, Felix Weltsch, and Robert Klopstock. And he finally leaves a woman (Ottla) with the task of curing him of whatever his ailment might be, thereby reversing the traditional gender politics of hysteria therapy.

Kafka's disavowals thus point ultimately beyond a fear of femininity – towards a complex understanding of the problem of medical diagnosis itself, especially its legal ramifications. The insurance industry's continued insistence on a single "determinate" or "principal" cause (*wesentliche Ursache*) conditioned Kafka's professional life, especially after the resuscitation of the medical-legal battle over simulation during the 1916 War Conference of German Neurologists – as discussed in chapter 3 and, relating to Freud, in chapter 2. Kafka's literary interrogations moved him beyond the anatomo-clinical etiologists enumerated in my introduction: Virchow, Koch, and, in terms of hysteria, Charcot. His fiction recalls instead the newer medical-philosophical thinkers who criticized truisms about determinate causes and even causality itself. Already in 1898, the physician Friedrich Martius censured monocausality as well as all "etiological thinking," which he characterized as "naïve."[8] And the famous physiologist Max Verworn joined a now growing chorus of anti-etiological voices in 1908. He disparaged causality as a "mystical concept emanating from a primitive phase of human thinking."[9]

Kafka would have known of such scepticism through his profession and through the writings of Ernst Mach, the world-famous physicist, philosopher, and physiologist at the University of Prague when Kafka was enrolled there. Mach criticized the "fetishistic" nature of causality as it had governed philosophical thinking since Kant.[10] This provided vital impulses to Einstein, who, later in life, embraced aspects of an anti-causal position close to the romantic image of *Zusammenhang* that I discussed in my introduction.[11] Kafka's fictional destruction of causality leans in this direction, yet with an added medical-legal twist stemming from his interest in the problem of insurance. Kafka's experiments surpassed those even of the most sophisticated medical thinkers of his day, who, as discussed in my introduction, allowed for "multiple" and "agglutinated" causalities and even for replacing causality with "conditionalism" (Verworn).[12] Yet they could not admit the full ramifications of this concession. For this would have catapulted diagnostics out of the world of insurance and compensation – as Martius writes, out of all "social legislation."[13] And this problem would have been especially complex for the traumatic neuroses.

The best contemporaneous corollary to Kafka's fiction is, fittingly, an unwittingly ironic one: Berlin Privy Counsellor Knoll's 1929 lecture to doctors about how to simplify insurance claims stemming from "accident and war neuroses." Knoll warns against the dangers of thinking too much about the philosophical problem of the "determinate cause." He mockingly asks: If there are determinate causes to modernity's ills should there not also be "non-determinate causes" (*nicht-wesentliche Ursachen*)? And might these not better be referred to as "preconditions" or "circumstances"? Instead of following this thought to its logical, legally impossible end, in which nearly every twentieth-century subject could be deemed ill, Knoll reminds doctors that the law insists that there *is* a "determinate cause." And that each judge will ascertain this as best he can, using his "common sense."[14] Kafka, with his sharp understanding of such contradictions, creates characters who *do* think this problem through to its end – just as Kafka does for his own phobia in 1922. Like one of his own characters, Kafka insists that his singular "physical" cause has become "mental" and, within this subgroup, blurred into a seemingly endless substitutive series. His phobia now seems to result from a plurality of causes so diverse in form and function as to resist causality itself. Kafka can ultimately describe the source only as the impossibly diffuse "fear in general."

Kafka's elucidation of this crisis of causality intensifies after the 1916 public debates in Munich on simulation, when Kafka's characters begin to understand "on their own bodies" Gregor Samsa's earlier complaints about the office gossip that a travelling salesman must endure: He suffers "on his own person [on his own body, *am eigenen Leibe*] the grim consequences, which can no longer be traced back to their causes [*Ursachen*]" (M 18, D 136–7). Kafka's late characters submit themselves to "government doctors" or to their substitutes for interpretation, but these examiners, even if they are benevolently inclined, always hit a diagnostic impasse. As was the case with the "little woman," they cannot localize "the causes of her condition." Kafka's characters subsequently gain neither social sympathy nor legal recourse. The narrators of "A Little Woman" and "Josefine, the Singer," speaking for the communal body of insurance, likewise assume that the protagonists are faking, but they can never tell for sure. The country doctor, an *Amtsarzt*, uniquely offers his patient a source, but this source appears dubious even to the patient. Gregor similarly did not know, already in 1912, if he was simulating, admitting that the suspicious *Kassenarzt* would not "be so very wrong" in accusing him of malingering (M 6). Although we are meant to understand this remark ironically (Gregor accepts every slander about him as true), the fact that he cannot adequately read his own body's signs gets to the core of the simulation quandary.

For even if Kafka's characters are simulating, they could still be ill, as some of Freud's colleagues argued even before Freud. Consider the work of the neurologist and psychiatrist Paul Julius Möbius, whom Freud considered one of the forefathers of psychoanalysis. Möbius asserted already in 1891 that, as in "First Distress," a person's thoughts or "ideas," including the very desire to be ill, could themselves be illnesses.[15] In 1906 the neurologist Ernst Bloch claimed that many signs of simulation mimicked exactly the signs of hysteria – especially the telltale "shaking" (*Zittern*) – such that distinguishing between the two was often a fool's errand.[16] This overlapping of simulation and illness culminated historically in an absurd-sounding early twentieth-century form of neurosis: the "Rentenneurose" (pension neurosis), caused apparently by the more or less conscious desire to receive a neurosis pension. With the *Rentenneurose*, the institution of social insurance that employed Kafka for most of his life came full circle: it was at once cure and cause. Kafka's 1916–17 simulator of death, the Hunter Gracchus, insists on this circularity: "The thought of wanting to help me is a sickness and requires bed rest" (K 112).

The zenith of such system-immanent pathologies was the *Rentenneurose*'s successor, the "Rentenkampfneurose" (pension-struggle neurosis), in which the fight to prove that one was truly ill likewise resulted itself in a neurosis. When the historian of science Greg Eghigian calls this phenomenon "Kafkaesque," he does not know how right he is. A neurotic suffering from "accusations of malingering," "countless medical exams," and "years of preoccupation with defending one's claim in court" does not merely recall, as Eghigian says, a Kafkan battle with bureaucracy in *The Trial* or *The Castle*.[17] More importantly, this "pension-struggle neurotic" is "Kafkaesque" because he battles to uncover a material origin that he will never be able to locate. We recall here Josefine in her "struggle" for "Anerkennung": meaning both "recognition" for her art (the usual translation) and, in the legal jargon that Kafka knew, the "acceptance of validity" of her pension claims. The ultimate cause of her neurasthenia remains unclear because she makes her "petitions" (*Forderungen*) based not on external circumstances but on "an inner logic" (K 105, D 372). This inner logic is that of the pension-struggle neurotic who cannot find a physical origin for her illness. She no longer knows: Is she ill because she is ill? Or because she desires to be recognized as ill? And what is the difference?

This pension-struggle neurotic becomes a model for Kafka's writing, which performs semiotically the same crisis of symptomatology. Symptoms are, for Kafka, "Krankheits-Zeichen," even though "Symptom," the borrowed Greek term, had been displacing the German "Krankheitszeichen" for almost a century.[18] Kafka's decision to employ this increasingly obsolete word draws attention to it, which further draws attention to the semiotic quandary at the heart of all symptoms. The symptom is a sign, Kafka insists, and moreover a tragic sign: it points to a substrate that is always missing. If this substrate can be found anywhere, it is only in the new social technology itself, which, as Kafka knew, had wanted to manage risk, accident, and shock, but found itself instead referring only back to its own origins. By creating an internal series of "nicht-wesentliche Ursachen," this insurance system inspired Kafka's aesthetic, which at once mirrored this system and ironized its attempt to pinpoint an etiology. Kafka tells us as much in his many statements about language, which recall Saussure's 1906 writings about the arbitrary nature of the linguistic sign. Language, like the medical sign of illness, cannot point to a truth. Rather, beyond the simplest matters in the "phenomenal world," language "can only be used allusively but never even approximately in a comparative way" (O 30).

Kafka presents language here as impoverished, as capable of speaking only obliquely. In so doing, he gives voice to the *Sprachkrise* (language crisis) that began with Kleist, Hoffmann, and the romantic ironists, then extended to Nietzsche, Mauthner, Rilke, Hofmannsthal, and Freud. Whereas some critics have claimed that this *Sprachkrise* was primarily "productive"[19] – a source of literary renewal – Kafka insists that it was not: Writing, he claims, is fully "helpless, cannot live in itself, is a joke and a despair" (Di 398). It can "merely attempt to say that the inconceivable is inconceivable," and as Kafka quips, "we knew that already" (K 161). He reacts in a vehemently non-"productive" way to language's crises, always dissatisfied with its ability to say what needs to be said. The best he can do is to construct a poetics of "indeterminacy," which remains "sheerly negative."[20]

This understanding of language as helpless might seem to disqualify Kafka's writing from saying anything about his historical epoch – specifically, as I have argued in this book, about his era's attempts to diagnose the traumas of modernity. Critics have drawn the obvious conclusion: Kafka's writing is an "allegory without historical power"; the "diachronic element" in his work is "entirely suppressed."[21] One might argue the same for E.T.A. Hoffmann and Freud, the other main figures that I have investigated. Hoffmann indeed claimed that writing transported him *away* from "external events," allowing him to create apparently timeless horror stories and fairy tales. And Freud often maintained that his theories were universal and non-diachronic: the Oedipus complex existed in ancient Greece exactly as it did in Vienna in 1900.

Beyond this, the styles of Hoffmann and Freud evince the same ineffability that we see in Kafka. Hoffmann peppers his texts with lacunae – ellipses and dashes – that suggest an inability to say the whole truth. Moreover, he relates the key scenes from "The Sandman" in free indirect style, letting the narrator's voice nearly disappear within that of Nathanael's – thereby disabusing us of the hope of an objective opinion. In *The Uncanny*, Freud similarly wavers uncertainly between first- and third-person perspectives, implying that uncanniness inheres precisely in the loss of this same outside point of view. There is no position from which to narrate authoritatively. Freud indeed spends most of the text telling us how hard it is to make a reliable statement about the "uncanny": he can define neither it nor the trauma that seems to cause it. This trauma eludes his investigations, here in *The Uncanny* and for the rest of his life.

Yet Freud's acknowledgment of his inability to identify the trauma at the source of uncanniness tells us something about the very diachrony that he, like Hoffmann and Kafka, otherwise suppresses. For this unintelligibility reveals traces of the unintelligible historical symptoms that all three writers will not – and, in some cases, cannot – represent. They reveal these to us through literary nuance and aporia. I think, first, of the traumatic style that Hoffmann transferred from his war diaries to "The Sandman." Through a blurring of perspective, he dramatizes the futile attempt to maintain an objective distance from trauma – at three levels: between his observing self and the war victims, between the narrator of "The Sandman" and Nathanael, and between himself and his own narrator from "The Sandman." This culminates in the story's ending, when the narrator, after witnessing the violent death of his friend, creates a brusque caesura through a dash that encompasses several years – a typographical symptom of repression that reminds us of Hoffmann's own experience in the war. Freud likewise abruptly breaks off his inconclusive investigations into the traumatic sources of uncanniness. In his final sentence from *The Uncanny*, he merely tells us that he has discussed these more fully "elsewhere," but he never tells us where, leaving us hanging, never able to locate this site of trauma (U 252). Hoffmann and Freud, like Kafka, gain their historical urgency through this indirectness. They do not use language straightforwardly to point or to refer. They decline to supply us with the missing "determinate cause."

For Kafka, writing can only tell the truth when it learns how not to do this, or at least how not to do so directly. This adds complexity to Kafka's famous remark about the relation of his task as a writer to the world around him. The writer must absorb and represent "the negative element" (*das Negative*) of this world. Kafka says, "I have vigorously absorbed the negative element of the age in which I live, an age that is, of course, very close to me, which I have no right ever to fight against, but as it were a right to represent." In order to represent the world's negative element, Kafka must adopt a negative form. As I have attempted to show in this book, he understands negative to mean not only "bad." He means also anti-positivistic (as in the causality debates) and also "negative" in the photographic sense. Kafka's job is to envision the world as a photographic negative (*das Negativ*) and thereby challenge positivism without forfeiting his right to represent the "age in which I live." He must say "no" to the revealed world and create images whose referents are present and absent at once. What was dark is light, and what was light is dark. Everything is reversed, ghostly, and barely recognizable – yet still there. Even Kafka's task itself, he insists, is actually only "the reflection of that task" (O 52, N2 98).

This indirectness and unnameability represent what we know to be the truth of trauma. It is both there and not there. The aesthetic that wants to record trauma must learn to express this absence without making it positively present. This kind of aesthetic – this poetics of trauma – ends up telling us the most we might hope to know about life in an era of shock, about what Freud, echoing Kafka, called in *The Uncanny* "the times in which we live." For as we have seen in Freud, Kafka, and Hoffmann, this poetics exposes, in negative form, the pathology at the heart of modernity: our insistence on finding a material source for all of our pathologies.

Notes

Introduction

1 Joyce, *Finnegans Wake*, 176.
2 Richard Ellmann, *James Joyce*, 386.
3 Spoo, "'Nestor' and the Nightmare," 138.
4 Barham, *Forgotten Lunatics*, 389n12. Other relatively recent scholars to connect *Ulysses* to World War I are Fairhall, who claims that the war "manifests itself as a ghostly future presence" in *Ulysses* (*James Joyce*, 168), and Birmingham, in *The Most Dangerous Book*, 52–3.
5 On World War I in Mann, Proust, and Joyce, see Beard, "Aesthetics of *Nachträglichkeit*."
6 See Cunliffe, "Cousin Joachim's Steel Helmet."
7 Middleton, "The Academic Development of *The Waste Land*," 171.
8 Maud Ellmann, "*The Waste Land*," 109 (see 101). See also Krockel, "Eliot's War Poetry."
9 Wolosky, *Emily Dickinson*, xviii.
10 Cixous, "La Fiction et ses fantômes," 199.
11 Oppenheim, *Die traumatischen Neurosen*, 125, 127. For more on Oppenheim and on the invention of the term "railway brain" by contemporaneous American scientists, see Fischer-Homberger, *Die traumatische Neurose*, 32–4; and Schivelbusch, *Geschichte der Eisenbahnreise*, 130–1.
12 Fischer-Homberger, *Die traumatische Neurose*, 24.
13 Fischer-Homberger, 24, 23.
14 Kleist, *Sämtliche Werke*, 4:634. On whether Kleist partially stages this "crisis," see Jochen Schmidt, *Kleist*, 12–16.
15 See Gauger, "Nietzsche," esp. 588–90.
16 Hofmannsthal, "Ein Brief," 49.
17 Saussure, *Course in General Linguistics*, 69.

18 Lévi-Strauss, *Marcel Mauss*, 63.
19 Koelb, *Kafka's Rhetoric*, 16.
20 On Kafka's legal-insurance work with veterans during the war, see Stach, *Jahre der Erkenntnis*, 78–90.
21 See Fischer-Homberger, *Die traumatische Neurose*, 56–73; and Lerner, *Hysterical Men*, 32–6.
22 Jünger, *In Stahlgewittern*, 15.
23 Micale, *Mind of Modernism*, 4–5.
24 Peset, "On the History of Medical Causality," 60–9.
25 Goetz, "Jean-Martin Charcot and the Anatomo-Clinical Method."
26 On Mach's (and William James's) reaction against positivism, see Ryan, *The Vanishing Subject*, 2. For Mach's critique specifically of John Stuart Mill's account of causality, see Mach, *Knowledge and Error*, 209–10.
27 Mach, *Knowledge and Error*, 205–6; *Erkenntnis und Irrtum*, 272–3. On Mach and "relation," see Russo, *Causality*, 8. On romantic *Zusammenhang* as a form of resisting logical causation, see (even if he incorrectly implies that Mach would have opposed *Zusammenhang*) Ben-Menahem, "Struggling with Causality," 303–4, 304n14.
28 See Ryan, *The Vanishing Subject*, 100–2 (Kafka), 115–23 (Hofmannsthal), 127–8 (Schnitzler), 208–17 (Musil). See also Corngold and Wagner, "Zarathustra on Laurentian Hill"; and Wilson, "Mach, Musil, and Modernism."
29 On the relation between Mach and the medical conditionalists, who resisted traditional causality, see Engelhardt, "Causality and Conditionality," 95n14. On the general critique of causality by Mach and medical researchers, see Fischer-Homberger, *Die traumatische Neurose*, 204–7.
30 Phelan, "*Fortgang* and *Zusammenhang*," 77 (see also 72).
31 Fischer-Homberger, *Die traumatische Neurose*, 206.

Chapter 1

1 On Hoffmann's escape into fantasy after Dresden, see Wührl, *E.T.A. Hoffmann*, 113. Steinecke finds such charges of "escapism" unfair but does admit that Hoffmann, in the period of *The Golden Pot*, aimed to move from "political happenings" towards the "poetic" ("Kommentar" in SW 2.1:748).
2 Drux's summary of the secondary literature on "The Sandman" makes no reference to the Battle of Dresden ("Die wissenschaftliche Rezeption"). A similar, more recent volume likewise contains no reference – even though it includes analyses from the perspectives of "New Historicism"

and "Psychoanalysis and Trauma Theory" (Jahraus, *Zugänge zur Literaturtheorie*, articles by Gerigk and Fricke, respectively). Breithaupt investigates Hoffmann's experiences of war and trauma but does not relate Dresden to his literary works ("Invention of Trauma"). Simon makes this relation but fails to mention "The Sandman," instead only "The Uncanny Guest" and "The Vow" ("Schlachtfeld, Stimmen"). Safranski similarly connects Dresden only to "The Uncanny Guest," "The Poet and the Composer," "The Elementary Spirit," and *The Magnetizer* (the latter predictively, for it was completed before the battle) (*Hoffmann*, 280–3, 294–6, 303, 309–10). In Engelstein's analysis of fragmented bodies, she notes cursorily that Hoffmann's experience of mutilated bodies in Dresden could have carried over to his description of Nathanael, but she does not investigate this (*Anxious Anatomy*, 176). Neumann comes closest, comparing Nathanael's shock to Freud's *The Uncanny* and then connecting Freud to World War I – but somehow still never mentioning Dresden ("Der Sandmann," 191).

3 Schelling, *Philosophie der Mythologie*, 515.
4 The Grimm dictionary locates only three isolated uses of *unheimlich* in the modern psychological sense of "dreadful, ghastly" before 1800 (*Deutsches Wörterbuch von Jacob und Wilhlem Grimm*, s.v. "unheimlich" 3 b, accessed Aug. 2, 2020, http://www.woerterbuchnetz.de/DWB ?lemma=unheimlich).
5 Although philosophers (Schelling, Marx, Nietzsche) mentioned uncanniness at the fringes of their work in the nineteenth century, the term only began to gain conceptual momentum in the early twentieth century. See Zilcosky, *Uncanny Encounters*, 17–18.
6 Castle, *The Female Thermometer*, 3–20.
7 Vidler, *The Architectural Uncanny*, 7–9.
8 Tolstoy, *War and Peace*, 1219.
9 For an overview of this literature, see Fricke, "ich war [...] von Coppelius gemisshandelt worden."
10 On Hoffmann's father abandoning him (when he was actually two years old), see Safranski, *Hoffmann*, 15–16.
11 For accounts of this Napoleonic era pathology by physicians during the Balkan Wars and World War I, see Laurent, *La guerre en Bulgarie*; and Anon., "Wind Contusions." For overviews, see Crocq and Crocq, "Shell Shock and War Neurosis," 48; Jones and Wessely, *Shell Shock to PTSD*, 2; and Jones, "Historical Approaches," 535. Another theory advanced during the Napoleonic Wars followed the long-standing claim that what we now call shell shock was caused by soldiers' "nostalgia" (Babington, *Shell Shock*, 8–9).

12 Dv 806 (*ängstlich*); Sg 19 (*Angst*); T 470 (*Wie wird's noch gehen!*).
13 On Rostov, see Rosenshield, "Trauma, Post-Traumatic Stress Disorder, and Recovery in *War and Peace*."
14 Tolstoy, *War and Peace*, 855, 931, 1187. See Freud SE 1:356, GW Nachtragsband: 448.
15 Although bits of free indirect style can be found in Renaissance, medieval, and even classical Greek texts, it emerges only as a continuous tradition in the early nineteenth century – in the works of Goethe, Austen, Büchner, and Hoffmann. See Pascal (who fails to include Hoffmann), *The Dual Voice*, 37–66.
16 The English translation sometimes adds quotation marks and italics where there are none, giving the false impression of narratorial intervention; it also omits the exclamation mark after "And yet!" (*Doch!*). I have corrected the translation accordingly.
17 Samuel Weber, *The Legend of Freud*, 17.
18 See Lacan, "Instance of the Letter in the Unconscious," 435–9.
19 See Braun, "Aspekte der Deutung," 81.
20 See Anhuber, *In einem fernen dunklen Spiegel*, 71.
21 See the editors' comments on this interrupted revision in SW 1:1337.
22 Hertz argued this first in "Freud and the Sandman." Others followed, including Noyes ("The Voice of History").
23 Hertz, "Freud and the Sandman," 310–13.
24 Hertz, 311–13.
25 See, for example, Sütterlin, "Phantom unseres eigenen Ichs," 97–8.
26 Fischer-Homberger, *Die traumatische Neurose*, 23, 24.

Chapter 2

1 The descriptions of 9/11 as "uncanny" are too numerous to list, but a sampling from the fields of cultural studies, psychology, and religion include Felix Hoffmann, *The Uncanny Familiar*; Connolly, "Psychoanalytic Theory"; and Heischman, "The Uncanniness of September 11th."
2 See Cixous, "La fiction et ses fantômes"; Samuel Weber "The Sideshow"; and Hertz, "Freud and the Sandman." For an overview of such 1970s articles, see Masschelein, *The Unconcept*, 95–131; and (from a critical perspective) Bartnæs, "Freud's 'The "Uncanny."'" On the potentially reactionary nature of such "anti-conceptualism," especially in the 1980s and onward, see Ffytche, "Night of the Unexpected."
3 Samuel Weber, "The Sideshow," 1132–3.
4 Vidler, *The Architectural Uncanny*, 7. Although Freud's essay (1919) was preceded by discussions of the uncanny by Ernst Jentsch (1906), Otto

Rank (1914), and Rudolf Otto (1917) (see Zilcosky, *Uncanny Encounters*, 17–18), Freud's is the only one to create a significant theoretical resonance – in, for example, Theodor Reik's *Der eigene und der fremde Gott* (1923), Edmund Bergler's "The Psycho-Analysis of the Uncanny" (1934), and the poststructuralist reaction in the wake of Derrida's "La double séance" (1970). Before Vidler, Gilbert and Gubar briefly related the term "uncanny" – albeit not actually Freud's essay – to soldiers' trench experiences (*No Man's Land*, 2:267).

5 Many later texts on *The Uncanny* (including Royle's *The Uncanny*) remain in the deconstructive tradition. On the continuation of this tradition into the 2000s, see Masschelein, *The Unconcept*, 1–2; for a criticism of this continuation's separation from the "particular" and from "historical context," see Ffytche, "Night of the Unexpected," 64–5.

6 Vidler, *The Architectural Uncanny*, 7.

7 Several scholars have restated Vidler's basic insight, yet none has fully enumerated Freud's observations about war and shock in *The Uncanny*. See the (brief) references in Rickels, *The Vampire Lectures*, 90; Royle, *The Uncanny*, 91; Wasson, *Urban Gothic*, 112; and Good, *Photography and September 11th*, 69. Bonikowski does not discuss *The Uncanny*, focusing instead on the "death drive" (*Shell Shock*). The only two scholars to discuss *The Uncanny* and the war in more than a cursory way, Haughton and Kaes, do not relate Freud's essay specifically to shell shock – even though shell shock is so central to Kaes's book (Haughton, "Introduction," lii–liii; Kaes, *Shell Shock Cinema*, 120–1).

8 Roe's explanation of why theosophy flourished in Australia during the war applies also to the other belligerent countries: mass death for "a noble cause created a bank of souls ready to incarnate for higher evolutionary purposes" (*Beyond Belief*, 225). As Winter writes, "the period of the 1914–1918 war was the apogee of spiritualism in Europe" (*Sites of Memory*, 76), even if, as Hazelgrove argues, spiritualist societies continued to grow in the decade or two afterwards (*Spiritualism and British Society*, 14–15). Haughton (Introduction to *The Uncanny*, liii) and Kaes (*Shell Shock Cinema*, 121) briefly connect this passage from *The Uncanny* to the postwar vogue for the occult.

9 Graves, *Goodbye to All That*, 192.

10 Lindsay, *My Mask*, 196.

11 Freud's patient, the Wolf-Man, claimed that Freud read Conan Doyle "attentively" (Gardiner, *The Wolf-Man*, 146). For more on Freud and Conan Doyle, see Marcus, Introduction to *Sherlock Holmes*, xi; Ginzburg, "Morelli, Freud and Sherlock Holmes"; and Brooks, *Reading for the Plot*, 269–70. On Conan Doyle's telepathy with his soldier son, see Winter, *Sites of Memory*, 58.

12 Mann attended his first séance in January, just two months after the
   armistice. Kurzke describes him as "almost" a believer (*Thomas Mann*,
   310; see 312–14).

13 Scapinelli, "Robert Reinert," 81.

14 Schoderer, "Geh bloß nicht in den Film!," 54. See also Kaes, who refers
   to the "uncanny telepathic relationship" between mother and son (*Shell
   Shock Cinema*, 41).

15 See the classic description by Remarque (*Im Westen*, 147–54) as well as
   Ernst Jünger's "unheimlich" experience of sleeping in a trench among
   French corpses (*In Stahlgewittern*, 33; see 18 for "unheimlich" French
   corpses). On the French side, René Nicolas sees in a captured German
   trench "dead piled upon dead, on the ground where you walked, above
   the parapets, in the walls of the trench, half buried, with either their
   heads sticking out or their feet or their hands or their knees" (*Campaign
   Diary*, 53). Cook cites these ever-present dead bodies – often used to reinforce trench walls – as a major source of the soldiers' belief in "ghosts,"
   the "uncanny," and the "return of the dead" ("Grave Beliefs").

16 Edmonds, *Military Operations*, 55.

17 Remarque, *Im Westen*, 75.

18 Jünger, *In Stahlgewittern*, 113, 302, 306.

19 Oppenheim, *Die Neurosen infolge von Kriegsverletzungen*, 196n1; for specific
   cases of *Verschüttung* see 9–10, 91–2, 95, 100–1, 104, 107–8, 114, 122,
   252–3; for further discussion of *Verschüttung*, see 210, 211.

20 Jünger, *In Stahlgewittern*, 73.

21 Ernst Simmel, *Kriegsneurosen*, 25. Although Simmel coined the term
   Verschüttungsneurose, many others connected *Verschüttung* to trauma.
   Wilhelm Schmidt likewise claimed that *Verschüttung* superseded grenade
   explosions as the major cause of shell shock ("Die psychischen und
   nervösen Folgezustände," 515); Birnbaum introduced the category of
   Verschüttungspsychose to his summary of wartime psychiatric research
   ("Kriegsneurosen und psychosen: Sammelbericht III," 345, 346); and
   even psychiatrists who believed that *Verschüttungstrauma* was faked used
   similar terms (Jolowicz's contribution to "Verhandlungen psychiatrischer
   Vereine," 208). For Freud's praise of Simmel's *Kriegsneurosen*, see Freud,
   Correspondence of Freud and Abraham, 372.

22 Ernst Simmel, "Zweites Korreferat," 45, 46; *Kriegsneurosen*, 25.

23 Ernst Simmel, "Zweites Korreferat," 47; see *Kriegsneurosen*, 25. Simmel
   uses *Verschüttung* as a psychological metaphor throughout both texts,
   most powerfully towards the end of *Kriegsneurosen*, when he refers to the
   traumatized soldier's "buried, weakened ego" (*das verschüttet gewesene*,

geschwächte Ich) (70). See also *Kriegsneurosen*, 39, 41, 50; and "Zweites Kor-referat," 48, 49, 51, 53.

24 Ernst Simmel, *Kriegsneurosen*, 15, 39, 11, 18, 24.

25 Hofmannsthal, *Der Schwierige*, 101. For a reading of *Der Schwierige* as a tale of *Verschüttungstrauma*, in the sense of both burial alive and ego submergence, see Mülder-Bach, "Herrenlose Häuser."

26 Kittler briefly mentions the connection between "Der Bau" and the wartime psychoanalytic discourse of *Verschüttung* – albeit without noticing Freud's own use of the term – in "Grabenkrieg," 299.

27 Moberly, "Inexplicable," 577. Despite the assiduous scholarly research into the texts Freud mentions in *The Uncanny*, "Inexplicable" has been neglected – absent even from a volume devoted specifically to Freud's reading (Gilman et al., *Reading Freud's Reading*). The only (brief) references to "Inexplicable" are by Quackelbeen and Nobus ("A propos de l'élucidation"); Lydenberg, ("Freud's Uncanny Narratives," 1082); Haughton (Introduction to *The Uncanny*, liii); Royle (*The Uncanny*, 135–40); and Iurascu ("Freud-the-Father").

28 Moberly, "Inexplicable," 581.

29 Moberly, 577.

30 Moberly, 578.

31 Moberly, 581.

32 On Freud's sons in the war, see Jones, *Freud*, 2:202–4.

33 Freud repeats the phrase "an der Leiche der geliebten Person" (beside the dead body of the loved one) on consecutive pages (GW 10:347, 348).

34 Freud, *Correspondence of Freud and Ferenczi*, 2:64. A few days after Freud's dream, Martin was indeed wounded on the Russian front (Gay, *Freud*, 354). For more on Freud's dreams about his soldier sons, see Jones, *Freud*, 2:180.

35 The few scholars to analyse this dream agree with Freud that it is primarily about death; none have noticed the dream son's resemblance to a shell-shock victim. See Lehmann, "Freud's Dream," and, for briefer treatments, Razinsky, *Freud*, 100–1, and Anzieu, *Freud's Self-Analysis*, 556.

36 For the typical symptoms of the war neurotic in World War I, see Fischer-Homberger, *Die traumatische Neurose*, 105–68; and Lerner, *Hysterical Men*, 61–85.

37 On the perceived similarity between epilepsy and shell shock, see Simmel, *Kriegsneurosen*, 6; and Smith and Pear, *Shell Shock*, 12.

38 This led, in the prelude to World War II, to the first experiments with acrylic eyes (Ott, "Hard Wear," 155–6).

39 Kienitz, "Die Kastrierten des Krieges," 70, 73.

40 Hirschfeld, *Sittengeschichte des Weltkrieges*, 46–7.
41 See Poore, *Disability*, 43–4; and Kaes, *Shell Shock Cinema*, 118–19.
42 See Gaupp's contribution to "Verhandlungen psychiatrischer Vereine," 203. For an overview of similar positions, see Lerner, *Hysterical Men*, 76.
43 This claim appeared in Walter Langer's confidential 1943 report to the CIA's predecessor, the OSS (declassified and published in 1972 as *The Mind of Hitler* [here, 156]). It is reasserted by Waite (*The Psychopathic God*, 204) and Binion (*Hitler among the Germans*, 5). Armbruster correctly notes that there are no primary documents supporting this diagnosis ("Behandlung Adolf Hitlers," 18–22).
44 Stekel, *Impotenz des Mannes*, 368, 390.
45 On the problems that the brute material event of technologized warfare posed for Freudian theory, see Malabou, *The New Wounded*, 77–161.
46 Ferenczi, "Die Psychoanalyse der Kriegsneurosen." Stekel and Abraham likewise focused on sexuality, albeit specifically on the return of repressed homosexual desires in the all-male world of the military. Although Simmel agreed with the psychoanalytic claim that shell shock revived infantile desires and anxieties, he de-emphasized sexuality (Stekel, *Impotenz des Mannes*, 373–8; Abraham, "Erstes Korreferat"; Simmel, *Kriegsneurosen* and "Zweites Korreferat"). For a review of the psychoanalytic responses to war neurosis, see Hirschfeld, *Sittengeschichte des Weltkrieges*, 64–9; and Lerner, *Hysterical Men*, 175–89. On Ferenczi, see Leys, *Trauma*, 138–47.
47 See Fischer-Homberger, *Die traumatische Neurose*, 77–82.
48 Oppenheim, *Die traumatischen Neurosen*, 125.
49 Cyrulnik cites chronic forms of "biological reaction" in children who live with traumatized parents (*Un merveilleux malheur*, 178). Schore argues that children in abusive "social-emotional environments" can experience long-term retardation of the brain's frontolimbic development ("Dysregulation of the Right Brain," 20). Yehuda speculates that PTSD results from the failure to curb a victim's "biologic stress response" at the moment of trauma ("Post-Traumatic Stress Disorder," 112).
50 Malabou, *The New Wounded*, 157.
51 Fischer-Homberger, *Die traumatische Neurose*, 16–101.
52 Leys connects these comments from *Beyond the Pleasure Principle* to Freud's economic theory of anxiety and primal repression in *Inhibitions, Symptoms and Anxiety* (*Trauma*, 21–35); Malabou expounds on the relation of these comments to the "narcissistic libido" from Freud's introduction to *Psycho-Analysis and the War Neuroses* (*The New Wounded*, 105–15).
53 See Lerner, *Hysterical Men*, 74–9, 137–9; and Fischer-Homberger, *Die traumatische Neurose*, 136–60.

54 Büttner, *Freud und der Erste Weltkrieg*, 95 (see his corresponding endnote 5 in the appendix).

55 Moberly, "Inexplicable," 578.

56 Moberly, 572.

57 Although Freud did not encourage his sons to fight, he also did not attempt to dissuade them when they (after being rejected or exempted from duty) chose to volunteer. On the exemption of Freud's sons and on his praise for Austria's "courageous" 1914 declaration of war, see Freud, *Correspondence of Freud and Abraham*, 265.

58 Moberly, "Inexplicable," 578, 579.

59 See Möbius, *Allgemeine Diagnostik*, 20, 208; and Eulenburg, *Encyclopädische Jahrbücher*, 102.

60 See Fischer-Homberger, *Die traumatische Neurose*, 16–168.

61 Freud writes of this "railway phobia" and his general "travel anxiety" (*Reiseangst*) – which he calls "my own hysteria" and once associated with seeing his mother naked in a train – in five separate 1897–9 letters. In addition to the three referred to in my main text, see F 268–9, 358; Fg 288–9, 393. Micale relates Freud's phobia to the same one in "Herr E.," whose five-year treatment was the longest undertaken by Freud in the nineteenth century (*Hysterical Men*, 260–5).

62 Singer, "Wesen und Bedeutung," 177 (also cited in Lerner, *Hysterical Men*, 41).

63 Lerner, 128.

64 Singer, "Prinzipien und Erfolge," 282.

65 Bonhoeffer, Expert Assessment of Eduard Meyer. As Bonhoeffer notes in this postwar assessment of Meyer (a "war hysteric"), doctors frequently used the term *Lazaretthysterie* (sometimes interchangeably with *Lazarettpsychose*) during the war. See Bonne, "Die Lazarettpsychose," 1192; and Birnbaum, "Kriegsneurosen und psychosen: Sammelbericht V," 205, and "Kriegsneurosen und psychosen: Sammelbericht VI," 31.

66 Cited in Eissler, *Freud as Expert Witness*, 47.

67 Lerner, *Hysterical Men*, 131–2.

68 R.A.E. Hoffmann describes wartime psychic "contagion" (*Ansteckung*) in "Über die Behandlung," 118. On psychic contagion generally, see Lerner, 70, 134–5.

69 Davoine and Gaudillière, *History beyond Trauma*, 49.

70 Caruth, *Trauma*, 10; *Unclaimed Experience*, 25. Leys criticizes Caruth for confounding victim and perpetrator, but Caruth rebuts with a complex relation of these two terms that includes, among other examples, the modern soldier betrayed by "the military or ruling class" (Leys, *Trauma*, 290–7; Caruth, *Unclaimed Experience*, 124).

71 Jünger, *In Stahlgewittern*, 15. Kaes connects this scene to the "allure of the occult," especially as depicted in Murnau's 1922 film *Nosferatu* (*Shell Shock Cinema*, 122).

72 Caruth, *Unclaimed Experience*, 129.

Chapter 3

1 Kafka, *Amerika: The Missing Person*, 101; *Der Verschollene*, 151.

2 Kafka, *Letters to Milena*, 223. On Kafka's fascination with this technological battle between "natural" and "ghostly" forces, see Zilcosky, *Kafka's Travels*, 153–73.

3 Max Maria von Weber, "Die Abnutzung des physischen Organismus," 228–9.

4 *Influence of Railway Travelling*, 41. For an overview of the early research on the railway's pathogenic shaking and inelasticity, see Schivelbusch, *Geschichte der Eisenbahnreise*, 106–13.

5 Wagner, "Simulation," 52.

6 Hirsch, "Reisekrankheiten," 301–2.

7 Reynolds, "Travelling: Its Influence on Health," 581.

8 Gotthilf, "Wie schützt man sich," 17. "Nervously predisposed" people should, Gotthilf claims, avoid the train's last, "especially swaying" car (18).

9 Hirsch cites Ernst Peters's *Vibrationsstuhl* as one of several possible cures for the two main kinetoses of his day: seasickness and railway neuroses ("Reisekrankheiten," 303).

10 Nordau, *Entartung*, 1:63, 66. Other late nineteenth- and early twentieth-century commentators likewise viewed neuroses as *Zivilisationskrankheiten* caused by railways (among other technologies) (Beard, *American Nervousness*, 112–13; Allbutt, "Nervous Disease," 214–21). For an overview, see Drinka, *Birth of Neurosis*, 108–22.

11 See Wagenbach, "Kafkas Fabriken," 26–31.

12 Corngold, *Necessity of Form*, 56, 76.

13 Among many such arguments, see Thiher, *Franz Kafka*, xi–xii, 33–50; Costa-Lima, *Limits of Voice*, 201–23; and Schuman, "Limits of Metaphorical Language."

14 The three most important early Kafka critics – Wilhelm Emrich, Heinz Politzer, and Walter Sokel – all made this claim, which continues to course through the secondary literature: Emrich, *Franz Kafka*, 115–27; Politzer, "Letter to His Father," 230; Sokel, *Tragik und Ironie*, 77–103.

15 On internal dialogues between specific Kafka texts, see Corngold, *Necessity of Form*, 228–49; and Anderson, *Kafka's Clothes*, 185–6. On Kafka's general intra-oeuvre communications, see Pasley, "Kafka's Semi-Private Games."

16 See Emrich, *Franz Kafka*, 127; and Binder, *Kafka-Kommentar*, 64.

17 On Kafka's business journeys, which became frequent beginning in 1908, see AS 981–6.

18 For contemporaneous theories of the "incubation period," see Erichsen, *Injuries of the Nervous System*, 74–5; Charcot, *Poliklinische Vorträge*, 99–100; and Freud, SE 1:52–3, 23:67. For overviews, see Schivelbusch, *Geschichte der Eisenbahnreise*, 123–6; Fischer-Homberger, *Die traumatische Neurose*, 110–11; Caruth, *Trauma*, 7; and Leys, *Trauma*, 19–20, 277–8.

19 Claudin, *Paris*, 73. Following a study of professional (train) travellers, one doctor claims never to have "seen any set of men so rapidly aged" (*Influence of Railway Travelling*, 53).

20 *Influence of Railway Travelling*, 40, 41, 53. For an overview of "fatigue" in railway travellers, see Schivelbush, *Geschichte der Eisenbahnreise*, 109–10, 113–16.

21 Erichsen, *Injuries of the Nervous System*, 76, 74. Not only crash victims but also people who simply caught "sight of a locomotive" or continually thought of "the possibility of collision" could develop neuroses (Schulze, *Die ersten deutschen Eisenbahnen*, 24; *Influence of Railway Travelling*, 43).

22 On these increases in speed, see Voigt, *Verkehr*, 1:865, 2:857 (on horse carriages). See also Voigt, 2:598; Radkau, *Zeitalter der Nervosität*, 193; and Kaschuba, *Überwindung der Distanz*, 174.

23 *Influence of Railway Travelling*, 44; Claudin, *Paris*, 72. In Kafka's day, doctors built on this particular aspect of Oppenheim's 1889 theory (see chapter 2): that severe railway vibrations or crashes caused a shrinking of the field of vision (see Wagner, "Simulation," 70). For more on the effects of railway travel upon vision, see Schivelbusch, *Geschichte der Eisenbahnreise*, 54–7.

24 Nordau, *Entartung*, 1:63.

25 Schnitzler, "Leutnant Gustl," 228. On the revolution in time caused by the railway in the second half of the nineteenth century, see Harrington, "Trains, Technology and Time-Travellers."

26 Winn, "Railway Traveling," 425.

27 Gotthilf, "Wie schützt man sich," 17, 18.

28 Hirsch, "Reisekrankheiten," 302.

29 Beicken summarizes early socio-critical interpretations of *The Metamorphosis* (*Kafka*, 265–6). See also Reimann, *Kafka aus Prager Sicht*; and Hughes, *Anthology of Marxist Criticism*.

30 Marx, *Kapital*, vol. 2 (*Marx Engels Werke* 24:160). My argument about Marx for the remainder of this paragraph follows Schivelbusch (*Geschichte der Eisenbahnreise*, 110–12).

31 Schivelbusch, 112.

32 In a letter to Felice Bauer, Kafka reports that he only travels third class (LF 530; see 186). See also Brod/Kafka, *Eine Freundschaft*, 191; and Stach, *Jahre der Erkenntnis*, 110.

33 Marx, *Kapital*, vol. 2 and vol. 1 (*Marx Engels Werke* 24:60, 23:445).

34 Cited in Schivelbusch, *Geschichte der Eisenbahnreise*, 187n8.

35 For an overview of the early criticism of *The Metamorphosis*, see Beicken, *Kafka*, 261–72; and Corngold, *Commentators' Despair*.

36 Santner, "Writing of Abjection," 298n8.

37 Gilman, *Jewish Patient*, 65, 80–1.

38 Corngold maintains that "the indeterminate, fluid crossing of a human tenor and a material vehicle is itself unsettling"; Gregor is an "opaque sign," a "mutilated metaphor, uprooted from familiar language" (*Necessity of Form*, 56, 59). Although arguing contra Corngold for the creative nature of this opacity, Koelb makes a similar point: the text's "indeterminacy" issues from the "possibility that signifiers" – such as the label of Gregor as "Ungeziefer" (vermin) – "might detach themselves from their immediate contextual limits" (*Kafka's Rhetoric*, 15, 16).

39 Psychiatrists intent on unmasking simulators often used this term, "work-shy" (*arbeitsscheu* or *arbeitsunlustig*), to describe apparent malingerers – for example, Cimbal, "Die seelischen und nervösen Erkrankungen," 414. See Lerner, *Hysterical Men*, 64–5.

40 On the introduction of railway liability laws, universal health insurance, and accident insurance in Germany, see Schäffner, "Event, Series, Trauma," 81–2; and Eghigian, "German Welfare State," 99–100. For the European context, see Micale, *Hysterical Men*, 140, 317n67.

41 The term "railway spine" has been credited to Erichsen, even though he tried to distance himself from it (*Injuries of the Nervous System*, 23). See Fischer-Homberger, "Railway Spine," and *Die traumatische Neurose*, 16–17.

42 Oppenheim, *Die traumatischen Neurosen*, 125, 127.

43 See Lerner, *Hysterical Men*, 32–3.

44 See Fischer-Homberger, *Die traumatische Neurose*, 56–73; and Lerner, *Hysterical Men*, 32–6.

45 Oppenheim, "Der Krieg und die traumatischen Neurosen," 257.

46 Cited in Fischer-Homberger, *Die traumatische Neurose*, 116.

47 See Fischer-Homberger, 73–83, 30.

48 For Freud's early (1895) claims regarding the importance of psychic predisposition, see SE 3:130–1. This theory becomes more central in his later work (SE 16:362, 18:31–2).

49 See Eghigian, "German Welfare State" (on West German legal changes in 1962), 110; and Schivelbusch, *Geschichte der Eisenbahnreise* (on British legal changes in 1963), 132.

50 Fischer-Homberger, *Die traumatische Neurose*, 23, 24.

51 Cited in Eissler, *Freud as Expert Witness*, 62.

52 Wagenbach, *In der Strafkolonie*, 77, 83–90 (new weaponry, planing machines); Kittler, "Schreibmaschinen, Sprechmaschinen," 116–41 (phonograph).

53 Taylor makes this classic argument in *War by Timetable*. See Westwood, *Railways at War*, 129; and Dennis Showalter, "Railroads and the German Way of War," 40.

54 Dennis Showalter, 21, 40.

55 Westwood, *Railways at War*, 122, 125, 129.

56 Mombauer, *Moltke*, 219. See Dennis Showalter, "Railroads and the German Way of War," 40; and Westwood, 131.

57 See Mombauer, 222.

58 On May 22, 1915, a British troop train collided with a civilian train, leaving at least 200 dead. On December 12, 1917, a French military train derailed; 543 soldiers were killed (Faith, *Derail*, 78–9).

59 The railway is, for Freud, the primary non-military cause of traumatic neuroses, as he emphasizes at his three major moments of discussing these neuroses: the late 1880s and early 1890s, when he reworks Charcot's theories of traumatic hysteria and develops his own; from 1917 to 1920, when he compares the railways to the war; and at the end of his life, in *Moses and Monotheism* and *Outline of Psychoanalysis*: SE 1:12 (1886); 1:51–2 (1888); 1:152 (1892); 16:274–5 (1917); 17:211–12 (1920); 18:12–13 (1920); 23:67–8 (1934–8); 23:184–5 (1938). See also SE 7:201–2 (1905) and 20:128 (1926).

60 Georg Simmel, "Metropolis," 410.

61 Benjamin, "Some Motifs in Baudelaire," 161–2.

62 Max Weber, "Die protestantische Ethik," 108.

63 Binder, *Kafkas "Verwandlung,"* 56–8, 67–76, 188–92, and 375–6 (for the biology book Kafka used in school, see 68 and 375).

64 *Deutsches Wörterbuch von Jacob Grimm und Wilhelm Grimm*, s.v. "Panzer," accessed Aug. 2, 2020, http://www.woerterbuchnetz.de/DWB?bookref =13,1428,22.

65 Binder, *Kafka-Kommentar*, 165.

66 See Hall, *Balkan Wars*, 136.

67 Stach, *Decisive Years*, 227.

68 Stach, 228–9.

69 From Brod's diary, cited in Stach, 229.
70 On the supposed brutality of the Montenegrins, see Hall, *Balkan Wars*, 136.
71 Remarque, *Im Westen*, 190.
72 On the German (Krupp) and French (Schneider-Creusot) weaponry used in the war, see Hall, *Balkan Wars*, 15–19.
73 Laurent, *La guerre en Bulgarie*. See Anon., "Wind Contusions"; and Roberts, *The Poison War*, 25–6. For an overview, see Jones and Wessely, *Shell Shock to PTSD*, 17–18.
74 Kafka indeed stops almost completely, with the meagre exceptions proving the rule: the "Blumfeld" fragment, a couple of pages of the never-completed "Assistant District Attorney," and seven lines of *Amerika* (Binder, *Kafka-Kommentar*, 190–2; Bezzel, *Kafka Chronik*, 103–22).
75 Many of these "shakers" were veterans, but some were not – just panhandlers who knew that twitching in borrowed uniforms increased their income (Lerner, *Hysterical Men*, 226–7).
76 Stach, *Jahre der Erkenntnis*, 78.
77 See Stach, 81, 80.
78 On Kafka's probable authorship of this article, which was signed by his boss, see AS 894–5.
79 On this article (and Kafka's second public appeal) as "war literature," see AS 81–4.
80 Fischer-Homberger, *Die traumatische Neurose*, 23.
81 See Lerner, *Hysterical Men*, 67–9.
82 Kaufmann, "Die planmäßige Heilung," 804.
83 On the relation between the simulation hunters and the Freudian "psychogenic" camp, see Fischer-Homberger, *Die traumatische Neurose*, 152–4; and Lerner, *Hysterical Men*, 187–9.
84 Cited in Eissler, *Freud as Expert Witness*, 62.
85 Remarque, *Im Westen*, 187–8.
86 Dr. Fritz Kaufmann's notorious "Kaufmann cure" gained wide acceptance during the war. See Lerner, *Hysterical Men*, 102–13; and Fischer-Homberger, *Die traumatische Neurose* 149–51.
87 See Stach, *Jahre der Erkenntnis*, 83–4.
88 On Freud's similar acceptance of "moderate" electrical treatment, see SE 17:213. On the outlawing of the high voltage "Kaufmann cure," see Stach, 630n26.
89 Stach, *Jahre der Erkenntnis*, 81 ("Invalidenrente"), 90 (on claims adjustment ["Regulierung"] and "negotiation").
90 Nordau, *Entartung*, 1:63, 68.

91 Because of this stereotype of hysteria as a feminine disorder, Charcot insisted that his male hysterics were virile, including a "manly artisan, solid, unemotional, a railway engineer." Cited in Elaine Showalter, "Hysteria, Feminism, Gender," 308–9.

92 On the male tendency to deny *Reiseangst* – specifically, "Eisenbahnangst" (railway-anxiety) – and displace it onto women, see Fischer-Homberger, *Die traumatische Neurose*, 41–2. On *Willensschwäche*, see Nordau, *Entartung*, 1:66; for an overview of this term at the fin de siècle, including its relation to hysteria and femininity, see Cowan, *Cult of the Will*, 10–15, 104–10, 269n61.

93 See Gilman, "Image of the Hysteric," 416–18, 405–6.

94 By the time Kafka wrote *The Metamorphosis*, his title was "Konzipist" (project manager). The important institutional "Prokura" (proxy power) had been granted to him on February 10, 1911 (AS 984). Kafka would never officially have been called "Prokurist" simply because governmental institutions like Kafka's did not use the term – even for someone who, like Kafka, had "Prokura" powers; I thank Benno Wagner for the latter point.

95 On the etymology of "Ungeziefer," see Corngold, *Necessity of Form*, 57.

96 Wagenbach, "Kafkas Fabriken," 31–40.

97 See Corngold, *Necessity of Form*, 54–5.

98 See AS 79–80; Stach, *Decisive Years*, 501, and *Jahre der Erkenntnis*, 81.

99 Engel and Robertson, preface to *Kafka, Prag und der Erste Weltkrieg*, 13–14.

100 The narrator of the one-paragraph story, "A Comment" (1922), says that he is on his way to a railway station, but the station is never described. The protagonist of "A Report to an Academy" (1917) rides on a steamship, but this was no longer particularly modern; the first diesel-powered ships, which were the death knell for the steamers, had appeared already in 1903.

101 The crossed-out section would belong on page 382 of Kafka, N1; for the facsimiled manuscript pages, see Kafka, *Oxforder Oktavheft 4*, 65–6.

102 Cited in Eissler, *Freud as Expert Witness*, 62.

103 On Kafka's literalizing strategy and suspicion of metaphor, see Corngold, *Necessity of Form*, 49–55.

104 For Kafka's statements about this representational crisis and its relation to his poetics, see Steele, "Kafka on Parables and Metaphors"; Corngold, *Necessity of Form*, 37–8, 51–7, 76–7, 149–50; and Koelb, *Kafka's Rhetoric*, 7–17.

105 See Heller, "Naturheilkunde contra Schulmedizin."

106 Kafka, *The Castle*, 145–6.

107 Stach, *Jahre der Erkenntnis*, 567.

108 The word *Graben* appears repeatedly in "Der Bau," but only the first English translators (Willa and Edwin Muir), working just over a quarter century after the war, rendered it accurately as "trench," albeit not consistently (sometimes as "hole," "excavation," "burrow," or "channel"). Later translators, more distanced from the war, have tended to use primarily "tunnel," even though Kafka never deploys the German cognate, "*Tunnel.*" Kittler demonstrates the relation of "Der Bau" to Kafka's work with injured veterans and trench warfare in "Grabenkrieg," 289–309.

109 Wilhelm Schmidt, "Die psychischen und nervösen Folgezustände," 515; see also Encke, *Augenblicke*, 128–51.

110 The major English translators (the Muirs, Pasley, Corngold) misleadingly render *Erdverschüttung* as "landslide," which would be "Erdrutsch" in German (see K 186). An *Erdrutsch* is only one possible cause of an *Erdverschüttung*, not the *Erdverschüttung* itself.

111 See Eghigian, "German Welfare State," 106.

112 For the Muir and Corngold translations, see CS 372, 374, 371 and K 104, 106, 104.

113 See Anderson, *Kafka's Clothes*, 194–216; Hermsdorf, "Künstler und Kunst," 95–7; and Fingerhut, *Die Funktion der Tierfiguren*, 292.

114 Corngold, *Necessity of Form*, 56; Koelb, *Kafka's Rhetoric*, 16.

115 Contemporaneous German texts that diagnosed the fin de siècle as the "age of nervousness" include Georg Simmel's above-mentioned "Die Großstädte und das Geistesleben" (1903), Karl Lamprecht's *Zur jüngsten deutschen Vergangenheit* (1902), Willy Hellpach's *Nervosität und Kultur* (1902), and Johannes Marcinowski's *Nervosität und Weltanschauung* (1910). For overviews, see Steiner, *Das nervöse Zeitalter*; Radkau, *Zeitalter der Nervosität*; Killen, *Berlin Electropolis*; and Cowan, *Cult of the Will*.

Conclusion

1 See Fischer-Homberger's subchapter on the "undetectable pathological-anatomical substrate" (*Die traumatische Neurose*, 23–6).

2 O'Connor and Drebing estimate that, at most, 35 per cent of veterans with brain injuries develop PTSD ("Veterans and Brain Injury," 175).

3 Peset, "On the History of Medical Causality," 70.

4 Nordau, *Entartung*, 1:66.

5 Wagner, "Simulation," 48. See Gotthilf, "Wie schützt man sich," 18; Conrad, "Eisenbahn und Gesundheit," 952; Hirsch, "Reisekrankheiten," 302.

6 On the relation of this fantasy streetcar to the one that Samsa's family boards at the end of *The Metamorphosis*, see Zilcosky, "Samsa war Reisender," 195–6.

7 Freud insists on the secrecy of Wilhelm Fliess, who has "witnessed one of my finest attacks of travel anxiety" – saying "this must remain strictly between us" (F, 358, 262).

8 Martius, "Krankheitsursachen und Krankheitsanlage," 93.

9 Verworn, *Frage nach den Grenzen der Erkenntnis*, 17.

10 Cited in Martius, "Das Kausalproblem," 101.

11 On Einstein and *Zusammenhang*, see Ben-Menahem, "Struggling with Causality," 303–4.

12 On Verworn and conditionalism, see Engelhardt, "Causality and Conditionality," 83–92.

13 Martius, "Das Kausalproblem," 125.

14 Cited in Fischer-Homberger, *Die traumatische Neurose*, 207.

15 Möbius, "Weitere Bemerkungen über Simulation," 679.

16 Bloch, "Einiges über die Simulation," 570.

17 Eghigian, "German Welfare State," 106.

18 The Greek-based "Symptom" displaced synonymous German medical terms in the course of the nineteenth century. *Deutsches Wörterbuch von Jacob Grimm und Wilhlem Grimm*, s.v. "Symptom," accessed Aug. 2, 2020, http://www.woerterbuchnetz.de/DWB?lemma=symptom.

19 Arens, "Linguistic Skepticism," 154.

20 Corngold, *Necessity of Form*, 57. Corngold marshals enough evidence from Kafka's diaries, journals, and stories to persuade us that Kafka indeed suffered from "the internal incoherence" of language and did *not* believe, as Gray et al. claim, in "the power to express one's thoughts perfectly" and to make "feelings expressed in words" correspond to those existing "in one's own heart" (*Kafka Encyclopedia*, 176–7).

21 Corngold, 149.

Works Cited

Abraham, Karl. "Erstes Korreferat." In Freud et al., *Psychoanalyse der Kriegsneurosen*, 31–41.

Allbutt, Clifford. "Nervous Disease and Modern Life." *Contemporary Review* 67 (1895): 210–31.

Anderson, Mark. *Kafka's Clothes: Ornament and Aestheticism in the Habsburg Fin de Siècle*. Oxford: Oxford University Press, 1992.

Anhuber, Friedhelm. *In einem fernen dunklen Spiegel: E.T.A. Hoffmanns Poetisierung der Medizin*. Opladen: Westdeutscher Verlag, 1986.

Anonymous. "Wind Contusions." *Lancet* 183, no. 4733 (16 May 1914): 1423.

Anzieu, Didier. *Freud's Self-Analysis*. London: Hogarth, 1986.

Arens, Katherine. "Linguistic Skepticism: Toward a Productive Definition." *Monatshefte* 74, no. 2 (1982): 145–55.

Armbruster, Jan. "Die Behandlung Adolf Hitlers im Lazarett Pasewalk 1918." *Journal für Neurologie, Neurochirurgie und Psychiatrie* 10 (2009): 18–22.

Babington, Anthony. *Shell Shock: A History of the Changing Attitudes to War Neurosis*. Barnsley: Pen & Sword, 2003.

Barham, Peter. *Forgotten Lunatics of the Great War*. New Haven: Yale University Press, 2004.

Bartnæs, Morten. "Freud's 'The "Uncanny"' and Deconstructive Criticism." *Psychoanalysis and History* 12, no. 1 (January 2010): 29–54.

Beard, George. *American Nervousness, Its Causes and Consequences: A Supplement to Nervous Exhaustion (Neurasthenia)*. New York, 1881.

Beard, Lauren. "The Aesthetics of *Nachträglichkeit*: Traumatic Temporality and the First World War in Proust, Joyce, and Mann." PhD diss., University of Toronto, 2020.

Beicken, Peter. *Franz Kafka: Eine kritische Einführung in die Forschung*. Frankfurt am Main: Athenaion, 1974.

Benjamin, Walter. "On Some Motifs in Baudelaire." In *Illuminations*, edited by Hannah Arendt, 155–200. New York: Schocken, 1969.

Ben-Menahem, Yemima. "Struggling with Causality: Einstein's Case." *Science in Context* 6, no. 1. (Spring 1993): 291–310.

Bezzel, Chris. *Kafka Chronik.* Munich: Hanser, 1975.

Binder, Hartmut. *Kafka-Kommentar zu sämtlichen Erzählungen.* Munich: Winkler, 1975.

– *Kafkas "Verwandlung": Entstehung, Deutung, Wirkung.* Frankfurt am Main: Stroemfeld, 2004.

Binion, Rudolph. *Hitler among the Germans.* New York: Elsevier, 1976.

Birmingham, Kevin. *The Most Dangerous Book: The Battle for James Joyce's "Ulysses."* London: Head of Zeus, 2014.

Birnbaum, Karl. "Kriegsneurosen und psychosen auf Grund der gegenwärtigen Kriegsbeobachtungen: Sammelbericht III." *Zeitschrift für die gesamte Neurologie und Psychiatrie: Referate und Ergebnisse* 12 (1916): 317–88.

– "Kriegsneurosen und psychosen auf Grund der gegenwärtigen Kriegsbeobachtungen: Sammelbericht V." *Zeitschrift für die gesamte Neurologie und Psychiatrie: Referate und Ergebnisse* 14 (1917): 193–258, 313–51.

– "Kriegsneurosen und psychosen auf Grund der gegenwärtigen Kriegsbeobachtungen: Sammelbericht VI." *Zeitschrift für die gesamte Neurologie und Psychiatrie: Referate und Ergebnisse* 16 (1918): 1–78.

Bloch, Ernst. "Einiges über die Simulation bei der traumatischen Neurose." *Medizinische Klinik* 2 (1906): 535–7, 568–70.

Bonhoeffer, Karl. Expert Assessment (*Gutachten*) of Eduard Meyer. 3 March 1922. File 23. Charité Nervenklinik Bestand. Humboldt University Archives, Berlin, Germany.

Bonikowski, Wyatt. *Shell Shock and the Modernist Imagination: The Death Drive in Post-World War I British Fiction.* Farnham: Ashgate, 2013.

Bonne, G.H. "Die Lazarettpsychose und ihre Verhütung." *Münchner medizinische Wochenschrift* 63 (December 1916): 1191–2.

Braun, Peter. "Aspekte der Deutung." In *Der Sandmann,* by E.T.A. Hoffmann, 72–81. Frankfurt am Main: Suhrkamp BasisBibliothek, 2003.

Breithaupt, Fritz. "The Invention of Trauma in German Romanticism." *Critical Inquiry* 32, no. 1 (Autumn 2005): 77–101.

Brod, Max, and Franz Kafka. *Eine Freundschaft,* edited by Malcolm Pasley. Vol. 1. Frankfurt am Main: Fischer: 1987.

Brooks, Peter. *Reading for the Plot.* New York: Knopf, 1984.

Büttner, Peter. "Freud und der Erste Weltkrieg: Eine Untersuchung über die Beziehung von medizinischer Theorie und gesellschaftlicher Praxis der Psychoanalyse." PhD diss., Ruprechts-Karls-Universität Heidelberg, 1975.

Caruth, Cathy, ed. *Trauma: Explorations in Memory.* Baltimore: Johns Hopkins University Press, 1995.

– *Unclaimed Experience: Trauma, Narrative, History.* 20th anniversary ed. Baltimore: Johns Hopkins University Press, 2016.

Castle, Terry. *The Female Thermometer: Eighteenth-Century Culture and the Invention of the Uncanny.* Oxford: Oxford University Press, 1995.

Charcot, Jean-Martin. *Poliklinische Vorträge (Leçons du mardi).* Vol. 1. Translated by Sigmund Freud. Leipzig, 1892.

Cimbal, Walter. "Die seelischen und nervösen Erkrankungen seit der Mobilmachung." *Neurologisches Zentralblatt* 34, no. 11 (1 June 1915): 411–15.

Cixous, Hélène. "La fiction et ses fantômes: Une lecture de l'*Unheimliche* de Freud." *Poétique* 10 (1972): 199–216.

Claudin, Gustave. *Paris.* Paris: Faurc, 1867.

Connolly, Angela. "Psychoanalytic Theory in Times of Terror." *Journal of Analytic Psychology* 48, no. 4 (September 2003): 407–31.

Conrad, M. "Einsenbahn und Gesundheit." *Reclams Universum* 2 (1902): 950–3.

Cook, Tim. "Grave Beliefs: Stories of the Supernatural and the Uncanny among Canada's Great War Trench Soldiers," *Journal of Military History* 77, no. 2 (April 2013): 521–42.

Corngold, Stanley. *The Commentators' Despair: The Interpretation of Kafka's "Metamorphosis."* Port Washington, NY: Kennikat, 1973.

– *Franz Kafka: The Necessity of Form.* Ithaca: Cornell University Press, 1988.

Corngold, Stanley, and Benno Wagner. "Zarathustra on Laurentian Hill: Quételet, Nietzsche, and Mach." In *Franz Kafka: The Ghosts in the Machine,* 17–33. Evanston: Northwestern University Press, 2011.

Costa-Lima, Luiz. *The Limits of Voice: Montaigne, Schlegel, Kafka.* Translated by Paulo Henriques Britto. Stanford: Stanford University Press, 1996.

Cowan, Michael. *Cult of the Will: Nervousness and German Modernity.* State College: Pennsylvania State University Press, 2008.

Crocq, Marc-Antoine, and Louis Crocq. "From Shell Shock and War Neurosis to Posttraumatic Stress Disorder: A History of Psychotraumatology." *Dialogues in Clinical Neuroscience* 2, no. 1 (March 2000): 47–55.

Cunliffe, W.G. "Cousin Joachim's Steel Helmet: *Der Zauberberg* and the War." *Monatshefte* 68, no. 4. (Winter 1976): 409–17.

Cyrulnik, Boris. *Un Merveilleux Malheur.* Paris: Odile Jacob, 1999.

Davoine, Françoise, and Jean-Max Gaudillière. *History beyond Trauma.* New York: Other Press, 2004.

Drinka, George Frederick. *The Birth of Neurosis: Myth, Malady, and the Victorians.* New York: Simon and Schuster, 1984.

Drux, Rudolf. "Die wissenschaftliche Rezeption." In *E.T.A. Hoffmann: Der Sandmann: Erläuterungen und Dokumente,* 78–118. Stuttgart: Reclam, 1994.

Edmonds, James. *Military Operations: France and Belgium, 1917.* Vol. 2. London: HMSO, 1948.

Eghigian, Greg. "The German Welfare State as a Discourse of Trauma." In Micale and Lerner, *Traumatic Pasts,* 92–112.

Eissler, Kurt. *Freud as an Expert Witness: The Discussion of War Neuroses between Freud and Wagner-Jauregg.* Translated by Christine Trollope. Madison, CT: International University Press, 1986.

Ellmann, Maud. "*The Waste Land*: A Sphinx without a Secret." In *The Poetics of Impersonality: T.S. Eliot and Ezra Pound,* 91–113. Cambridge, MA: Harvard University Press, 1987.

Ellmann, Richard. *James Joyce.* Revised ed. Oxford: Oxford University Press, 1982.

Emrich, Wilhelm. *Franz Kafka.* Frankfurt am Main: Athenäum, 1965.

Encke, Julia. *Augenblicke der Gefahr: Der Krieg und die Sinne.* Munich: Fink, 2006.

Engel, Manfred, and Ritchie Robertson, eds. *Kafka, Prag und der Erste Weltkrieg.* Würzburg: Königshausen & Neumann, 2012.

Engelhardt, Dietrich von. "Causality and Conditionality in Medicine around 1900." In *Science, Technology, and the Art of Medicine,* edited by Corinna Delkeskamp-Hayes and Mary Ann Gardell Cutter, 75–104. Dordrecht: Kluwer, 1993.

Engelstein, Stefani. *Anxious Anatomy: The Conception of the Human Form in Literary and Naturalist Discourse.* Albany: SUNY Press, 2008.

Erichsen, John Eric. *On Railway and Other Injuries of the Nervous System.* Philadelphia, 1867.

Eulenburg, Albert. *Encyclopädische Jahrbücher der gesammten Heilkunde.* Vienna, 1891.

Fairhall, James. *James Joyce and the Question of History.* Cambridge: Cambridge University Press, 1993.

Faith, Nicholas. *Derail: Why Trains Crash.* London: Macmillan, 2000.

Ferenczi, Sándor. "Die Psychoanalyse der Kriegsneurosen." In Freud et al., *Psychoanalyse der Kriegsneurosen,* 9–30.

Ffytche, Matt. "Night of the Unexpected: A Critique of the 'Uncanny' and Its Apotheosis within Cultural and Social Theory." *New Formations* 75 (Spring 2012): 63–81.

Fingerhut, Karl-Heinz. *Die Funktion der Tierfiguren im Werke Franz Kafkas: Offene Erzählgerüste und Figurenspiele.* Bonn: Bouvier, 1968.

Fischer-Homberger, Esther. "Railway Spine und traumatische Neurose – Seele und Rückenmark." *Gesnerus* 27, no. 1/2 (1970): 96–111.

– *Die traumatische Neurose: Vom somatischen zum sozialen Leiden.* Gießen: Psychosozial-Verlag, 2004.

Freud, Sigmund. *Briefe an Wilhelm Fließ 1874–1904.* Edited by Jeffrey Moussaieff Masson. Frankfurt am Main: Fischer, 1986.

– *The Complete Correspondence of Sigmund Freud and Karl Abraham 1907–1925.* Edited by Ernst Falzeder. London: Karnac, 2002.

– *The Complete Letters of Sigmund Freud to Wilhelm Fliess, 1887–1904.* Edited by Jeffrey Moussaieff Masson. Cambridge, MA: Harvard Univ. Press, 1985.

– *The Correspondence of Sigmund Freud and Sándor Ferenczi.* Edited by E. Brabant, E. Falzeder, and P. Giampieri-Deutsch. 3 vols. Cambridge, MA: Harvard University Press, 1993–2000.

– *Gesammelte Werke.* Edited by Anna Freud et al. 19 vols. London: Imago, 1940–87.

– *The Standard Edition of the Complete Psychological Works.* Edited and translated by James Strachey. 24 vols. London: Hogarth Press & the Institute of Psychoanalysis, 1953–74.

Freud, Sigmund, Sándor Ferenczi, Karl Abraham, Ernst Simmel, and Ernest Jones. *Zur Psychoanalyse der Kriegsneurosen.* Leipzig: Internationaler Psychoanalytischer Verlag, 1919.

Fricke, Hannes. "'ich war […] von Coppelius gemisshandelt worden': Literaturpsychologische Zugangsweisen am Beispiel von Psychoanalyse und Traumatheorie." In Jahraus, *Zugänge zur Literaturtheorie*, 177–96.

Gardiner, Muriel, ed. *The Wolf-Man by the Wolf-Man.* New York: Basic Books, 1971.

Gauger, Hans-Martin. "Nietzsche: Zur Genealogie der Sprache." In vol. 1 of *Theorien vom Ursprung der Sprache*, edited by Joachim Gessinger and Wolfert von Rahden, 585–606. Berlin: de Gruyter, 1988.

Gay, Peter. *Freud: A Life for Our Time.* New York: Norton, 1998.

Gerigk, Anja. "Verhandlungen mit Hoffmanns Sandmann: Eine Repräsentationsanalyse des Interieurs im 19. Jahrhundert als neuhistorische Praxis." In Jahraus, *Zugänge zur Literaturtheorie*, 138–48.

Gilbert, Sandra, and Susan Gubar. *No Man's Land: The Place of the Woman Writer in the Twentieth Century.* 3 vols. New Haven: Yale University Press, 1988–96.

Gilman, Sander. *Franz Kafka: The Jewish Patient.* New York: Routledge, 1995.

– "The Image of the Hysteric." In Gilman et al., *Hysteria beyond Freud*, 345–452.

Gilman, Sander, Jutta Birmele, Jay Geller, and Valerie Greenberg, eds. *Reading Freud's Reading.* New York: New York University Press, 1994.

Gilman, Sander, Helen King, Roy Porter, G.S. Rousseau, and Elaine Showalter. *Hysteria beyond Freud.* Berkeley: University of California Press, 1993.

Ginzburg, Carlo. "Morelli, Freud and Sherlock Holmes." *History Workshop* 9 (1980): 5–36.

Goetz, Christopher. "Jean-Martin Charcot and the Anatomo-Clinical Method of Neurology." *Handbook of Clinical Neurology* 95 (December 2009): 203–12.

Good, Jennifer. *Photography and September 11th: Spectacle, Memory, Trauma.* London: Bloomsbury, 2015.

Gotthilf, Otto. "Wie schützt man sich beim Eisenbahnfahren gegen Gesundheitsschädigungen." *Deutsche Alpenzeitung* 1, no. 9 (1901/2): 17–18.

Graves, Robert. *Goodbye to All That.* Harmondsworth: Penguin, 1960.

Gray, Richard, Ruth Gross, Rolf Goebel, and Clayton Koelb. *A Franz Kafka Encyclopedia.* Westport, CT: Greenwood, 2005.

Hall, Richard C. *The Balkan Wars 1912–1913: Prelude to the First World War.* New York: Routledge, 2000.

Harrington, Ralph. "Trains, Technology and Time-Travellers: How the Victorians Re-Invented Time." Artificial Horizon, 2003. https://www.yumpu .com/en/document/view/46933189/trains-technology-and-time-travellers -artificialhorizon.org.

Haughton, Hugh. Introduction to *The Uncanny* by Sigmund Freud, lii–liii. Translated by David McLintock. London: Penguin, 2003.

Hazelgrove, Jenny. *Spiritualism and British Society between the Wars.* Manchester: Manchester University Press, 2000.

Heischman, Daniel. "The Uncanniness of September 11th." *Journal of Religion and Health* 41, no. 3 (September 2002): 197–205.

Heller, Paul. "Naturheilkunde contra Schulmedizin: 'Ein Landarzt.'" In *Franz Kafka: Wissenschaft und Wissenschaftskritik*, 92–102. Tübingen: Stauffenburg, 1989.

Hermsdorf, Klaus. "Künstler und Kunst bei Franz Kafka." In Reimann, *Kafka aus Prager Sicht*, 95–106.

Hertz, Neil. "Freud and the Sandman." In *Textual Strategies: Perspectives in Post-Structuralist Criticism*, edited by Josué Harari, 296–321. Ithaca: Cornell University Press, 1979.

Hirsch, Max. "Reisekrankheiten." *Therapeutische Rundschau* 2, no. 19 (10 May 1908): 301–4.

Hirschfeld, Magnus, ed. *Sittengeschichte des Weltkrieges.* Vol. 2. Leipzig: Verlag für Sexualwissenschaft, 1930.

Hoffmann, E.T.A. *Sämtliche Werke.* Edited by Hartmut Steinecke and Wulf Segebrecht. 6 vols. Frankfurt am Main: Deutscher Klassiker Verlag, 1985–2004.

– *Tales of Hoffmann.* Translated by R.J. Hollingdale. London: Penguin, 1982.

Hoffmann, Felix, ed. *The Uncanny Familiar: Images of Terror.* Cologne: König, 2011.

Hoffmann, R.A.E. "Über die Behandlung der Kriegshysterie in den badischen Nervenlazaretten." *Zeitschrift für die gesamte Neurologie und Psychiatrie* 55, no. 1 (December 1920): 114–47.

Hofmannsthal, Hugo von. "Ein Brief." In *Sämtliche Werke: Kritische Ausgabe*, edited by Rudolf Hirsch, Clemens Köttelwesch, Heinz Rölleke, and Ernst Zinn, 31:45–55. Frankfurt am Main: Fischer, 1975–.

– *Der Schwierige: Lustspiel in drei Akten.* In *Sämtliche Werke*, 12:5–144.

Hughes, Kenneth, ed. *Franz Kafka: An Anthology of Marxist Criticism.* Hanover: University Press of New England, 1981.

The Influence of Railway Travelling on Public Health. London, 1862.

Iurascu, Ilinca. "Freud-the-Father, Ernst-the-Son." Paper presented at the NeMLA Convention, Philadelphia, March 2006.

Jahraus, Oliver, ed. *Zugänge zur Literaturtheorie: 17 Modellanalysen zu E.T.A. Hoffmanns "Der Sandmann."* Stuttgart: Reclam, 2016.

Jay, Martin. "The Uncanny Nineties," *Salmagundi* 108 (Fall 1995): 20–9.

Jones, Edgar. "Historical Approaches to Post-Combat Disorders." *Philosophical Transactions: Biological Sciences* 361, no. 1468 (April 2006): 533–42.

Jones, Edgar, and Simon Wessely. *Shell Shock to PTSD: Military Psychiatry from 1900 to the Gulf War.* New York: Psychology Press, 2005.

Jones, Ernest. *The Life and Work of Sigmund Freud.* 3 vols. New York: Basic Books, 1953–7.

Joyce, James. *Finnegans Wake.* New York: Viking, 1939.

Jünger, Ernst. *In Stahlgewittern.* Hamburg: Deutsche Hausbücherei, 1926. First published 1920.

Kaes, Anton. *Shell Shock Cinema: Weimar Culture and the Wounds of War.* Princeton: Princeton University Press, 2009.

Kafka, Franz. *Amerika: The Missing Person.* Translated by Mark Harman. New York: Schocken, 2008.

– *Amtliche Schriften.* Edited by Klaus Hermsdorf and Benno Wagner. Frankfurt am Main: Fischer, 2004.

– *The Blue Octavo Notebooks.* Translated by Ernest Kaiser and Eithne Wilkins. Cambridge, MA: Exact Change, 1991.

– *Briefe 1902–1924.* Edited by Max Brod. Frankfurt am Main: Fischer, 1958.

– *Briefe an Felice.* Edited by Erich Heller and Jürgen Born. Frankfurt am Main: Fischer, 1967.

– *The Castle.* Translated by Mark Harman. New York: Schocken, 1998.

– *The Complete Stories.* Edited by Nahum Glatzer. New York: Schocken, 1971.

– *Diaries 1910–23.* Edited by Max Brod. New York: Schocken, 1976.

– *Drucke zu Lebzeiten.* Edited by Hans-Gerd Koch, Wolf Kittler, and Gerhard Neumann. Frankfurt am Main: Fischer, 1994.

– *Kafka's Selected Stories.* Translated by Stanley Corngold. New York: Norton, 2007.

– *Letters to Felice.* Translated by James Stern and Elisabeth Duckworth. New York: Schocken, 1973.

– *Letters to Friends, Family, and Editors.* Translated by Richard Winston and Clara Winston. New York: Schocken, 1977.

– *Letters to Milena.* Translated by Philip Boehm. New York: Schocken, 1990.

- *The Metamorphosis.* Translated and edited by Stanley Corngold. New York: Modern Library, 2013.
- *The Metamorphosis, the Penal Colony, and Other Stories.* Translated by Willa and Edwin Muir. New York: Schocken, 1975.
- *Nachgelassene Schriften und Fragmente.* 2 vols. Edited by Malcolm Pasley (vol. 1) and Jost Schillemeit (vol. 2). Frankfurt am Main: Fischer, 1992–3.
- *Oxforder Oktavheft 4.* In *Historisch-Kritische Ausgabe.* Edited by Roland Reuß and Peter Staengle. Frankfurt am Main: Stroemfeld, 2008.
- *Der Verschollene.* Edited by Jost Schillemeit. Frankfurt am Main: Fischer, 1983.
Kaschuba, Wolfgang. *Die Überwindung der Distanz: Zeit und Raum in der europäischen Moderne.* Frankfurt am Main: Fischer, 2004.
Kaufmann, Fritz. "Die planmäßige Heilung komplizierter psychogener Bewegungsstörungen bei Soldaten in einer Sitzung." *Münchener medizinischer Wochenschrift* 63 (1916): 802–4.
Kienitz, Sabine. "Die Kastrierten des Krieges: Körperbilder und Männlichkeitskonstruktionen im und nach dem Ersten Weltkrieg." *Zeitschrift für Volkskunde* 95 (1999): 63–82.
Killen, Andreas. *Berlin Electroplis: Shocks, Nerves, and German Modernity.* Berkeley: University of California Press, 2005.
Kittler, Wolf. "Grabenkrieg – Nervenkrieg – Medienkrieg: Franz Kafka und der 1. Weltkrieg." In *Armaturen der Sinne: Literarische und technische Medien 1870 bis 1920,* edited by Jochen Hörisch and Michael Wetzel, 289–309. Munich: Fink, 1990.
- "Schreibmaschinen, Sprechmaschinen: Effekte technischer Medien im Werk Franz Kafkas." In *Franz Kafka, Schriftverkehr,* edited by Kittler and Gerhard Neumann, 75–163. Freiburg: Rombach, 1990.
Kleist, Heinrich von. *Sämtliche Werke und Briefe.* Edited by Helmut Sembdner. 4 vols. Munich: Hanser, 1982.
Koelb, Clayton. *Kafka's Rhetoric: The Passion of Reading.* New York: Cornell University Press, 1989.
Krockel, Carl. "Eliot's War Poetry: 'Hysteria' to *The Waste Land.*" In *War Trauma and English Modernism: T.S. Eliot and D.H. Lawrence,* 89–127. New York: Palgrave, 2011.
Kurzke, Hermann. *Thomas Mann: Life as a Work of Art.* Princeton: Princeton University Press, 2002.
Lacan, Jacques. "The Instance of the Letter in the Unconscious, or Reason Since Freud." In *Écrits,* translated by Bruce Fink, 412–41. New York: Norton, 2006.
Langer, Walter. *The Mind of Hitler: The Secret Wartime Report.* New York: Basic Books, 1972.

Laurent, Octave. *La guerre en Bulgarie et en Turquie: Onze mois de campagne.* Paris: A. Maloine, 1914.

Lehmann, Herbert. "Freud's Dream of February 1918." *International Review of Psycho-Analysis* 10 (1983): 87–93.

Lerner, Paul. *Hysterical Men: War, Psychiatry, and the Politics of Trauma in Germany, 1890–1930.* Ithaca: Cornell University Press, 2003.

Lévi-Strauss, Claude. *Introduction to the Work of Marcel Mauss.* Translated by Felicity Baker. London: Routledge & Kegan Paul, 1987.

Leys, Ruth. *Trauma: A Genealogy.* Chicago: University of Chicago Press, 2000.

Lindsay, Norman. *My Mask: For What Little I Know of the Man behind It; An Autobiography.* Sydney: Angus and Robertson, 1970.

Lydenberg, Robin. "Freud's Uncanny Narratives." *PMLA* 112, no. 5 (October 1997): 1072–86.

Mach, Ernst. *Erkenntnis und Irrtum: Skizzen zur Psychologie der Forschung.* Leipzig: J.A. Barth, 1905.

– *Knowledge and Error: Sketches on the Psychology of Enquiry.* Vol. 3 of Vienna Circle Collection. With an introduction by Erwin N. Hiebert. Dordrecht: D. Reidel, 1976.

Malabou, Catherine. *The New Wounded: From Neurosis to Brain Damage.* Translated by Steven Miller. New York: Fordham University Press, 2012.

Marcinowski, Johannes. *Nervosität und Weltanschauung.* Berlin: O. Salle, 1910.

Marcus, Steven. Introduction to *The Sherlock Holmes Illustrated Omnibus,* by Arthur Conan Doyle. New York: Schocken, 1976.

Martius, Friedrich. "Das Kausalproblem in der Medizin." *Beihefte zur Medizinischen Klinik* 5 (1914): 101–28.

– "Krankheitsursachen und Krankheitsanlage." *Verhandlungen der Gesellschaft deutscher Naturforscher und Ärzte* 70 (September 1898): 90–110.

Marx, Karl. *Das Kapital: Kritik der politischen Ökonomie.* 3 vols. Vols. 23–5 of *Marx Engels Werke.* Berlin: Dietz, 1962–4.

Masschelein, Anneleen. *The Unconcept: The Freudian Uncanny in Late Twentieth-Century Theory.* Albany: SUNY Press, 2011.

Micale, Marc. *Hysterical Men: The Hidden History of Male Nervous Illness.* Harvard University Press, 2008.

–, ed. *The Mind of Modernism: Medicine, Psychology, and the Cultural Arts in Europe and America, 1880–1940.* Stanford: Stanford University Press, 2004.

Micale, Marc, and Paul Lerner, eds. *Traumatic Pasts: History, Psychiatry, and Trauma in the Modern Age, 1870–1930.* Cambridge: Cambridge University Press, 2001.

Middleton, Peter. "The Academic Development of *The Waste Land.*" In *Demarcating the Disciplines: Philosophy Literature Art,* edited by Samuel Weber, 153–80. Minneapolis: University of Minnesota Press, 1986.

Moberly, L.G. "Inexplicable." *Strand Magazine* 54 (1917): 572–81.

Möbius, P.J. *Allgemeine Diagnostik der Nervenkrankheiten.* Leipzig: Vogel, 1886.

– "Weitere Bemerkungen über Simulation bei Unfall-Krankheiten." *Münchener medizinische Wochenschrift* 38 (1891): 677–80.

Mombauer, Annika. *Helmuth von Moltke and the Origins of the First World War.* Cambridge: Cambridge University Press, 2001.

Mülder-Bach, Inka. "Herrenlose Häuser: Das Trauma der Verschüttung und die Passage der Sprache in Hofmannsthals Komödie 'Der Schwierige.'" In *Hugo von Hofmannsthal: Neue Wege der Forschung,* edited by Elsbeth Dangel-Pelloquin, 162–85. Darmstadt: Wissenschaftliche Buchgesellschaft, 2007.

Neumann, Gerhard. "Der Sandmann." In *Meisterwerke der Literatur: Von Homer bis Musil,* edited by Reinhard Brandt, 185–226. Stuttgart: Reclam, 2001.

Nicolas, René. *Campaign Diary of a French Officer.* New York: Houghton Mifflin, 1917.

Nordau, Max. *Entartung.* 2 vols. Berlin: Duncker, 1892–3.

Noyes, John. "The Voice of History: Sigmund Freud/E.T.A. Hoffmann/ G.H. Schubert." *Journal of Literary Studies* 6, nos. 1–2 (1990): 36–61.

O'Connor, Maureen, and Charles Drebing. "Veterans and Brain Injury." In *Living Life Fully after Brain Injury,* edited by Robert Fraser, Kurt Johnson, and Kathleen Bell, 171–93. Youngsville, NC: Lash & Associates, 2011.

Oppenheim, Hermann. "Der Krieg und die traumatischen Neurosen." *Berliner klinische Wochenschrift* 52 (15 March 1915): 257–61.

– *Die Neurosen infolge von Kriegsverletzungen.* Berlin: Karger, 1916.

– *Die traumatischen Neurosen nach den in der Nervenklinik der Charité in den letzten 5 Jahren gesammelten Beobachtungen.* Berlin, 1889.

Ott, Katherine. "Hard Wear and Soft Tissue: Craft and Commerce in Artificial Eyes." In *Artificial Part, Practical Lives: Modern Histories of Prosthetics,* edited by Katherine Ott, David Serlin, and Stephen Mihm, 147–70. New York: New York University Press, 2002.

Pascal, Roy. *The Dual Voice: Free Indirect Speech and Its Functioning in the Nineteenth-Century European Novel.* Manchester: Manchester University Press, 1977.

Pasley, Malcolm. "Kafka's Semi-Private Games." *Oxford German Studies* 6, no. 1 (1971): 112–32.

Peset, José Luis. "On the History of Medical Causality." In *Science, Technology, and the Art of Medicine,* edited by Corinna Delkeskamp-Hayes and Mary Ann Gardell Cutter, 57–74. Dordrecht: Kluwer, 1993.

Phelan, Anthony. "*Fortgang* and *Zusammenhang*: Walter Benjamin and the Romantic Novel." In *Walter Benjamin and Romanticism,* edited by Andrew Benjamin and Beatrice Hanssen, 69–82. New York: Continuum, 2002.

Politzer, Heinz. "Letter to His Father." In *Franz Kafka Today*, edited by Angel Flores and Homer Swander, 221–37. Madison: University of Wisconsin Press, 1964.

Poore, Carole. *Disability in Twentieth-Century German Culture*. Ann Arbor: University of Michigan Press, 2007.

Quackelbeen, Julien and Dany Nobus. "A propos de l'élucidation d'une reference freudienne: L'*Inexplicable* de L.G. Moberly." *Quarto* 48/9 (1992): 83–7.

Radkau, Joachim. *Das Zeitalter der Nervosität: Deutschland zwischen Bismarck und Hitler*. Munich: Hanser, 1998.

Razinsky, Liran. *Freud, Psychoanalysis and Death*. Cambridge: Cambridge University Press, 2013.

Reimann, Paul, ed. *Franz Kafka aus Prager Sicht*. Berlin: Voltaire, 1966.

Remarque, Erich Maria. *Im Westen nichts Neues*. Cologne: Kiepenheuer & Witsch, 1998. First published 1929.

Reynolds, J. Russell. "Travelling: Its Influence on Health." In *The Book of Health*, edited by Malcolm Morris, 559–88. London, 1884.

Rickels, Laurence A. *The Vampire Lectures*. Minneapolis: University of Minnesota Press, 1999.

Roberts, A. A. *The Poison War*. London: William Heinemann, 1915.

Roe, Jill. *Beyond Belief: Theosophy in Australia 1879–1939*. Sydney: UNSW Press, 1986.

Rosenshield, Gary. "On Trauma, Post-Traumatic Stress Disorder, and Recovery in *War and Peace*: The Case of Nikolai Rostov." *Tolstoy Studies Journal* 25 (2013): 22–41.

Royle, Nicholas. *The Uncanny*. Manchester: Manchester University Press, 2003.

Russo, Federica. *Causality and Causal Modelling in the Social Sciences: Measuring Variations*. Vol. 5 of *Methodos Series: Methodological Prospects in the Social Sciences*. Dordrecht: Springer, 2009.

Ryan, Judith. *The Vanishing Subject: Early Psychology and Literary Modernism*. Chicago: University of Chicago Press, 1991.

Safranski, Rüdiger. *E.T.A. Hoffmann: Das Leben eines skeptischen Phantasten*. 2nd ed. Frankfurt am Main: Fischer, 2000.

Santner, Eric. "Kafka's *Metamorphosis* and the Writing of Abjection." In Kafka, *The Metamorphosis*, 223–44, 298–302 (endnotes).

Saussure, Ferdinand de. *Course in General Linguistics*. Translated by Wade Baskin. New York: Philosophical Library, 1959.

Scapinelli, Karl Graf. "Bei Robert Reinert." *Deutsche Lichtspiel-Zeitung* no. 28 (19 July 1919): 81–2.

Schäffner, Wolfgang. "Event, Series, Trauma: The Probabilistic Revolution of the Mind in the Late Nineteenth and Early Twentieth Centuries." In Micale and Lerner, *Traumatic Pasts*, 81–91.

Schelling, Friedrich Wilhelm Joseph. *Philosophie der Mythologie.* 5th supplemental vol. of *Schellings Werke,* edited by Manfred Schröter. Munich: Beck, 1968.

Schivelbusch, Wolfgang. *Geschichte der Eisenbahnreise: Zur Industrialisierung von Raum und Zeit im 19. Jahrhundert.* Munich: Hanser, 1977.

Schmidt, Jochen. *Heinrich von Kleist: Die Dramen und Erzählungen in ihrer Epoche.* Darmstadt: Wissenschaftliche Buchgesellschaft, 2003.

Schmidt, Wilhelm. "Die psychischen und nervösen Folgezustände nach Granatexplosionen und Minenverschüttungen." *Zeitschrift für die gesamte Neurologie und Psychiatrie* 29, no. 1 (December 1915): 514–42.

Schnitzler, Arthur. "Leutnant Gustl." In *Gesammelte Werke in Einzelausgabe: Das erzählerische Werk,* 2:207–36. Frankfurt am Main: Fischer Taschenbuch Verlag, 1984.

Schoderer, Julia. "'Geh bloß nicht in den Film, der ist dermaßen aufregend!' Zur sinnlichen Inszenierung moderner Krisenphänomene im Stummfilm am Beispiel von Robert Reinerts *Nerven.*" In *Anschauen und Vorstellen: Gelenkte Imagination im Kino,* edited by Heinz-Peter Preußer, 52–67. Marburg: Schüren, 2014.

Schore, Allan. "Dysregulation of the Right Brain: A Fundamental Mechanism of Traumatic Attachment and the Psychopathogenesis of Posttraumatic Stress Disorder." *Australian and New Zealand Journal of Psychiatry* 36, no. 1 (May 2002): 9–30.

Schulze, F.K.A. *Die ersten deutschen Eisenbahnen.* 2nd ed. Leipzig: Voigtlander, 1917.

Schuman, Rebecca. "Kafka's *Verwandlung,* Wittgenstein's *Tractatus,* and the Limits of Metaphorical Language." *Modern Austrian Literature* 44, no. 3/4 (2011): 19–32.

Showalter, Dennis, E. "Railroads, the Prussian Army, and the German Way of War in the Nineteenth Century." In *Railways and International Politics: Paths of Empire, 1848–1945,* edited by T.G. Otte and Keith Neilson, 21–44. New York: Routledge, 2006.

Showalter, Elaine. "Hysteria, Feminism, Gender." In Gilman et al., *Hysteria beyond Freud,* 286–344.

Simmel, Ernst. *Kriegsneurosen und 'Psychisches Trauma': Ihre gegenseitigen Beziehungen dargestellt auf Grund psycho-analytischer, hypnotischer Studien.* Munich: Nemnich, 1918.

– "Zweites Korreferat." In Freud et al., *Psychoanalyse der Kriegsneurosen,* 42–60.

Simmel, Georg. "The Metropolis and Mental Life" ("Die Großstädte und das Geistesleben" [1903]). In *The Sociology of Georg Simmel,* translated by Kurt Wolff, 409–24. Glencoe: Free Press, 1950.

Simon, Ralf. "Schlachtfeld, Stimmen (E.T.A. Hoffmann)." *Colloquium Helveticum* 39 (2008): 179–96.

Singer, Kurt. "Prinzipien und Erfolge der aktiven Therapie bei Neurosen." *Zeitschrift für physikalische und diätetische Therapie* 22, no. 8/9 (Aug./Sept. 1918): 275–85.

Singer, Kurt. "Wesen und Bedeutung der Kriegspsychosen." *Berliner Klinische Wochenschrift* 52, no. 8 (22 Feb. 1915): 177–80.

Smith, G. Elliot, and T.H. Pear. *Shell Shock and Its Lessons.* London: Longmans, Green, 1917.

Sokel, Walter. *Franz Kafka: Tragik und Ironie.* Munich: Langen Müller, 1964.

Spoo, Robert. "'Nestor' and the Nightmare: The Presence of the Great War in *Ulysses.*" *Twentieth Century Literature* 32, no. 2. (Summer 1986): 137–54.

Stach, Reiner. *Kafka: The Decisive Years.* New York: Harcourt, 2005.

– *Kafka: Die Jahre der Erkenntnis.* Frankfurt am Main: Fischer, 2008.

Steele, Benjamin David. "Kafka on Parables and Metaphors, Writing and Language." *Marmalade* (blog). *Wordpress*, March 7, 2014. https://benjamindavidsteele.wordpress.com/2014/03/07/kafka-on-parables-and-metaphors-writing-and-language/.

Steiner, Andreas. *Das nervöse Zeitalter: Der Begriff der Nervosität bei Laien und Ärzten in Deutschland und Österreich um 1900.* Zurich: Juris, 1964.

Stekel, Wilhelm. *Die Impotenz des Mannes.* Vol. 4 of *Störungen des Trieb- und Affektlebens.* Berlin: Urban & Schwarzenberg, 1920.

Sütterlin, Nicole A. "'Phantom unseres eigenen Ichs' oder 'verfluchter Doppeltgänger?' Über die Unentscheidbarkeit von Hoffmanns *Der Sandmann.*" In Jahraus, *Zugänge zur Literaturtheorie,* 84–100.

Taylor, A.J.P. *War by Timetable: How the First World War Began.* London: MacDonald, 1969.

Thiher, Allen. *Franz Kafka: A Study of the Short Fiction.* Boston: Twayne, 1990.

Tolstoy, Leo. *War and Peace.* Revised and edited with an introduction by Amy Mandelker. Translated by Louise Maude and Aylmer Maude. Oxford: Oxford University Press, 2010.

"Verhandlungen psychiatrischer Vereine: Kriegstagung des Deutschen Vereins für Psychiatrie zu München." *Allgemeine Zeitschrift für Psychiatrie und psychisch-gerichtliche Medizin* 73 (1917): 163–233.

Verworn, Max. *Die Frage nach den Grenzen der Erkenntnis.* Jena: G. Fischer, 1908.

Vidler, Anthony. *The Architectural Uncanny.* Cambridge, MA: MIT Press, 1992.

Voigt, Fritz. *Verkehr.* Berlin: Duncker & Humblot, 1965–73.

Wagenbach, Klaus, ed. *In der Strafkolonie: Eine Geschichte aus dem Jahre 1914.* Expanded ed. Berlin: Wagenbach, 1995.

– "Kafkas Fabriken." In *Kafkas Fabriken,* edited by Hans-Gerd Koch and Klaus Wagenbach, 3–40. 2nd ed. Marbach: Deutsche Schillergesellschaft, 2003.

Wagner, Rudolf. "Simulation im Bahnbetriebe mit besonderer Berücksichtigung der sogenannten 'traumatischen Neurose.'" *Aerztliche Sachverständigen-Zeitung* 6 (1900): 47–52, 69–73.

Waite, Robert. *The Psychopathic God: Adolf Hitler.* New York: Basic Books, 1977.

Wasson, Sara. *Urban Gothic of the Second World War: Dark London.* New York: Palgrave, 2010.

Weber, Max. "Die protestantische Ethik und der 'Geist' des Kapitalismus (II): Die Berufsidee des asketischen Protestantismus." *Archiv für Sozialwissenschaft und Sozialpolitik* 21 (1905): 1–110.

Weber, Max Maria von. "Die Abnutzung des physischen Organismus beim Fahrpersonal der Eisenbahnen." *Wieck's Illustrirte Deutsche Gewerbezeitung* 25 (1860): 225–9.

Weber, Samuel. *The Legend of Freud.* Expanded ed. Stanford: Stanford University Press, 2000.

– "The Sideshow, or: Remarks on a Canny Moment." *MLN* 88, no. 6 (December 1973): 1102–33.

Westwood, John. *Railways at War.* San Diego: Howell-North, 1980.

Wilson, Catherine. "Mach, Musil, and Modernism." *The Monist* 97, no. 1. (January 2014): 138–55.

Winn, J.M. "Railway Traveling, and Its Effects on Health." *The Journal of Public Health, and Sanitary Review* 1, no. 4 (Dec. 1855): 425–6.

Winter, Jay. *Sites of Memory, Sites of Mourning: The Great War in European Cultural History.* Cambridge: Cambridge University Press, 2014.

Wolosky, Shira. *Emily Dickinson: A Voice of War.* Newhaven, CT: Yale University Press, 1984.

Wührl, Paul-Wolfgang. *E.T.A. Hoffmann: Der goldne Topf: Erläuterungen und Dokumente.* Stuttgart: Reclam, 1982.

Yehuda, Rachel. "Post-Traumatic Stress Disorder." *New England Journal of Medicine* 346, no. 2 (January 2002): 108–14.

Zilcosky, John. *Kafka's Travels: Exoticism, Colonialism, and the Traffic of Writing.* New York: Palgrave Macmillan, 2003.

– "'Samsa war Reisender': Trains, Trauma, and the Unreadable Body." In *Kafka for the Twenty-First Century,* edited by Stanley Corngold and Ruth Gross, 179–206. Rochester: Camden House, 2011.

– *Uncanny Encounters: Literature, Psychoanalysis, and the End of Alterity.* Evanston: Northwestern University Press, 2016.

Index

63; railways liable, 46, 82–3;
ruthless punctuality, 78–80, 86–7,
145n58; symptoms of, 71, 76–7,
81, 143n19, 143n21; texts chosen,
reasons for, 11–12; traumatic
neurosis, 46, 83–4, 87, 95, 145n59;
treatments for, 72, 142n9; war/
railway neuroses as contagious,
9, 10, 43, 57, 62–7, 108; without
railway or war trauma, 101–4,
106–9. *See also* Freud, Sigmund;
Kafka, Franz; shell shock
Remarque, Erich Maria, 45–6, 91,
97, 102
Rentenkampfneurose/pension-struggle
neurosis, 6, 128–9; *Rentenkampf/*
struggle for a pension, 113–14
Rilke, Rainer Maria, 7
romantic and modern literature
of trauma: categorization of, 15;
crisis in semiotics of traumatic
illness, 14–15, 81–3; language as
apparently non-referential, 39–40,
82–3, 84–5; language scepticism,
6–8, 15, 102, 118, 126–7; texts
chosen, reasons for, 11–12,
15; texts with hidden/missed
references, 4–6, 9–10, 21–2, 37–9,
42–3, 134–5n2, 137n7; traumatic
form of narration in, 9; uncanny,
use of term, 41–2. *See also* literary
criticism; *specific authors*
Rossmann, Karl, 69

Saussure, Ferdinand de, 8–9
Schelling, Friedrich Wilhelm Joseph,
22
Schivelbusch, Wolfgang, 80
Schnitzler, Arthur, 12–13;
"Lieutenant Gustl," 78, 91

semiotics of trauma: Kafka's poetics
of indeterminacy, 73–4, 100, 111–
12, 130, 132; language scepticism,
8–9, 102; medicine's semiotic
crisis, 10, 12, 14–15, 82–3, 102;
sign of illness (*Krankheitszeichen*),
8, 10, 102, 104, 108, 118, 129–30
sexuality and war neuroses, 59–61.
See also blindness and castration,
fear of; Freud, Sigmund
shell shock (war neurosis): diagnosis
of cerebro-medullary shock, 92;
electrical therapy, high voltage,
97–8; epilepsy and, 53–4; Kafka's
writing soliciting care for, 93–6,
100–1, 107; physical cause/
etiology, 57–8, 66–7, 84, 87–8,
92, 105–6, 123, 126, 128, 145n59;
predisposition, 124, 127–8;
soldiers' "nostalgia," 135n11; war
shakers/*Kriegszitterer*, 26–7, 46,
53–4, *54*, 57, 93–4, 141n65; war
shakers prefigured, 70–1; without
war or railway trauma, 101–4, 106–
9; World War I and, 5, 6, 42, 53–4,
58. *See also* burial/*Verschüttung*
and fear of live burial; simulation,
battle over/*Simulationsstreit*; World
War I
Simmel, Ernst, 46–7, 57–8, 87–8,
138n23
simulation, battle
over/*Simulationsstreit*: electrical
therapy, high voltage, 97–8;
insurance industry and trauma
diagnosis, 83–4, 121–2, 126,
144n39; in Kafka's writing,
10, 107–8, 112–18, 128;
Rentenkampfneurose/pension-
struggle neurosis, 6, 128–9; as

Milton Keynes UK
Ingram Content Group UK Ltd.
UKHW012227190424
441406UK00001B/118